Improving Healthcare

Good intentions to do our best in healthcare are not enough. Healthcare professionals need to know how to close the gap between best evidence and practice, by understanding and applying quality improvement principles and processes.

Improving Healthcare is a practical guide, providing healthcare staff with the knowledge and skills that enable them to implement, evaluate and disseminate a quality improvement project in their own workplace. With a comprehensive coverage, chapters cover the history, selection and application of quality improvement philosophies and methods in clinical healthcare at team, unit, organisational and system levels. The book also considers social processes of implementation as well as technical aspects of measuring and improving quality.

As an essential guide for healthcare practitioners at any level, *Improving Healthcare* includes practical examples and case studies of healthcare improvement that illustrate the concepts discussed.

Lesley Baillie is Florence Nightingale Foundation Chair of Clinical Nursing Practice in the School of Health and Social Care at London South Bank University.

Elaine Maxwell is Associate Professor in Leadership at London South Bank University.

Improving Healthcare
A Handbook for Practitioners

Edited by
Lesley Baillie and Elaine Maxwell

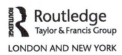
Routledge
Taylor & Francis Group

LONDON AND NEW YORK

First published 2017
by Routledge
2 Park Square, Milton Park, Abingdon, Oxon OX14 4RN

and by Routledge
711 Third Avenue, New York, NY 10017

Routledge is an imprint of the Taylor & Francis Group, an informa business

British Library Cataloguing-in-Publication Data
A catalogue record for this book is available from the British Library

---

Library of Congress Cataloging-in-Publication Data

Names: Baillie, Lesley, author. | Maxwell, Elaine, author.
Title: Improving healthcare : a handbook for practitioners / Lesley Baillie
and Elaine Maxwell.
Description: Abingdon, Oxon ; New York, NY : Routledge/Taylor & Francis
Group, 2017. | Includes bibliographical references.
Identifiers: LCCN 2016049346| ISBN 9781138709249 (hardback) | ISBN
9781498744461 (pbk.) | ISBN 9781315151823 (ebook)
Subjects: | MESH: Quality Assurance, Health Care—methods | Quality
Improvement | Outcome and Process Assessment (Health Care)
Classification: LCC R733 | NLM W 84.41 | DDC 610—dc23
LC record available at https://lccn.loc.gov/2016049346

ISBN: 978-1-4987-4446-1 (pbk)
ISBN: 978-1-138-70924-9 (hbk)
ISBN: 978-1-315-15182-3 (ebk)

Typeset in Sabon
by diacriTech

Table of Contents

Preface

In this book, we assert that good intentions to do our best in healthcare are not enough; healthcare professionals need to know how to close the gap between best evidence and practice, and between expected and actual outcomes through a better understanding of the principles and processes of employing quality improvement strategies. Quality improvement needs to be studied as rigorously and evidenced as comprehensively as clinical interventions. Practitioners who are able to think critically about the underpinning concepts of improvement are better able to apply them to their own workplace and are far more likely to bring about sustained improvements than those who would try to simply copy techniques that appear to have worked in other environments.

The aim of this book is therefore to provide frontline staff with the knowledge and skills to enable them to plan, implement, evaluate and disseminate quality improvement work in practice. The scope of the book covers the history, selection and application of quality improvement philosophies and methods in clinical healthcare at team, unit, organisational and system levels. This book considers social processes of implementation as well as technical aspects of measuring and improving quality. Each chapter begins with an introduction and objectives and provides a balance of theory with practical application and case study examples throughout.

Chapter 1 provides a history of quality in healthcare with early examples of how data has been used to demonstrate variation and measure improvement and an introduction to quality improvement methodologies that are in current use in healthcare. The chapter explains how approaches to improvement in manufacturing, which use a systems approach, rather than focusing on individual responsibility, have since been applied to healthcare. The change from a focus on quality control to quality improvement is examined, and an introduction to human factors and their application to safety in healthcare is provided.

Chapter 2 introduces context and explores the influences on improvement of the content of the change proposed, the context for improvement and the processes undertaken during improvement. The nature of culture and climate and their effects on improvement are also explored, with ethnography considered as a way of understanding the context for improvement. Organisational readiness for change and ways of assessing readiness are also explored, and there are examples of how contextual factors have affected quality improvements in practice.

Healthcare delivery is increasingly complex and involves multiple systems and so we need to understand the system in which care is provided when planning and implementing improvement work. Chapter 3 therefore focuses on systems theory with application to healthcare practice and improvement and includes a discussion of LEAN principles within the context of systems thinking. The chapter highlights how teams, as microsystems, play an essential role within improvement activity, as the larger system cannot otherwise improve.

Integration of microsystems and different types and levels of integration are reviewed in relation to healthcare delivery and improvement. Finally, the chapter examines interprofessional and collaborative working within systems and provides examples related to quality improvement in healthcare.

Chapter 4 discusses how service user involvement in quality improvement has evolved over recent years, and the innovative ways in which service and quality improvement projects can successfully involve service users in their design and delivery. The chapter considers how service user involvement in quality improvement can be evaluated, and includes practical case studies of service user involvement in improvement.

In Chapter 5, the institutional, professional and ethical duty to improve quality in healthcare is examined prior to an analysis of ethical considerations in quality improvement. This chapter applies the biomedical ethical principles of autonomy, non-maleficence, beneficence and justice to quality improvement, and approaches to ethical approval and governance in practice are then addressed. Finally, the ethical obligation to disseminate quality improvement work is considered.

The focus of Chapter 6 is on measurement in quality improvement. The chapter emphasises the importance of selecting an appropriate measurement plan during quality improvement, and the strengths and weaknesses of different approaches are examined. The chapter reviews different measurement tools and considers the use of metrics and dashboards, and statistical process control charts are also explained.

In Chapter 7, the theory of High Reliability Organisations (HROs) is examined in depth with application to healthcare improvement and how care can be made safer through reliability, resilience and organisational learning. The principles of risk analysis and risk control for enhancing reliability are explored and the importance of performance variability for enhancing resilience is explained. The chapter discusses the role of organisational learning for sustaining progress with patient safety and concludes by acknowledging that the journey towards becoming an HRO requires vision, leadership and an organisational culture of safety and improvement.

Knowing what best practice is and being able to implement best practice are two different activities and so the focus of Chapter 8 is on implementing improvement. Theories of change are explained and there is an examination of how developing a local theory of change model for a specific improvement can support implementation in practice. The chapter then proceeds to explore how quality improvement can be scaled up across multiple sites, and sustainability of improvement over time is also examined.

The dissemination of improvement work is essential and Chapter 9 provides an in-depth examination on ways to share and disseminate improvement work effectively. The chapter explains how to capture the essential information, ways of communicating improvement concurrently with the improvement work and how to write an effective improvement report. Planning for publication and dissemination is addressed and other approaches to sharing the work are included.

For quality improvement to be useful and create lasting change, evaluation must be an integral part of the improvement plan. Therefore, in Chapter 10, the nature of quality improvement evaluation is explored with an analysis of evaluation methodologies and associated strengths and limitations. The range of data sources that can be included in evaluations are discussed and ways of analysing the data are considered. The chapter emphasises that understanding the impact of quality improvement interventions is imperative for the refinement of the design and further improvement.

We hope that this book will make a valuable contribution to your learning and understanding of improvement in healthcare, which you can apply to your own areas to make positive changes in practice that are sustainable and will impact the quality of healthcare.

Lesley Baillie and Elaine Maxwell

Editors

Lesley Baillie, PhD, MSc, BSc (Hons), RN, is Florence Nightingale Foundation Chair in the School of Health and Social Care at London South Bank University (London, United Kingdom). Her post is held jointly with University College London Hospitals NHS Foundation Trust, and she is also the director of the Centre for Nurse and Midwife–led Research and an honorary professor at the University College London. Dr. Baillie has extensive experience in clinical practice, research and education and her research interests include improving quality of care, integrated care and dignity in care.

Elaine Maxwell, PhD, MSc, BA(Hons) RN, is an associate professor in leadership at London South Bank University. After a career in the NHS, including posts as executive director of nursing, she worked at the Health Foundation before moving into academia. Dr. Maxwell's interests include patient safety, quality improvement and professional role jurisdictions. She is a member of the editorial board of the *Journal of Research in Nursing*.

Contributors

Helen Crisp is an assistant director at the Health Foundation, overseeing grants to external researchers for research into quality improvement in healthcare. She is also working on translational research to put methods developed through health economics research to achieve better value for money in the allocation of healthcare budgets into practice in the National Health Service (NHS). Before joining the Foundation, Crisp spent 17 years working on healthcare quality accreditation, initially on the King's Fund Organisational Audit Programme, developing quality standards for hospital services, mental health, primary care and hospices.

Jerusha Murdoch Kelly, DipHE, RN (Child Branch), is the head of Nursing and Quality for Children and Young Peoples Services at Basildon and Thurrock University Hospitals NHS Foundation Trust. Kelly has been a paediatric nurse for over 20 years, working in a variety of settings including paediatric intensive care and acute paediatric wards.

Mark-Alexander Sujan, PhD, is an associate professor at Warwick Medical School (Coventry, United Kingdom), and has a background in safety and human factors and resilience engineering in a range of industries. Dr. Sujan holds a particular interest in proactive approaches to patient safety management, resilient healthcare systems and the transfer of safety engineering and human factors engineering knowledge across disciplines.

Nicola Thomas, RGN, BSc (Hons), MA, PhD, is an associate professor in Kidney Care, London South Bank University. Dr. Thomas has worked within the renal speciality for her entire career and her particular research interest is the self-management of kidney disease. She has been involved in two national quality improvement projects in the United Kingdom, funded by the Health Foundation. She is president of the European Dialysis and Transplant Nurses Association/European Renal Care Association (EDTNA/ERCA) and is the editor of the *Journal of Renal Care*.

Susan Went, MPH, MBA, MCSP, is the director of Nerissa Consulting Ltd. (London), providing consultancy to organisations and teams who want to implement change, improve their systems of care or build organisational improvement capacity and capability. Went holds a clinical qualification in physiotherapy and was previously the director of Evidence and Improvement, at Healthcare Improvement Scotland.

1 Introducing Healthcare Improvement

Elaine Maxwell

Introduction

Healthcare professionals choose their career out of a desire to do their best for other people and undertake rigorous training to ensure that they know what constitutes effective clinical care. The evidence threshold for clinical interventions is rightly set high, and most health-care professions across the world these days require graduate-level preparation. However, the long acknowledged gap between theory and practice persists despite many people's best efforts to close it. In addition, the gap between predicted and actual outcomes remains high. Every first-world country can point to examples of spectacular failures in healthcare, but per-haps less visible and more insidious are the variations in patient outcomes, and experiences within healthcare systems that are by and large performing acceptably. If we can get it right some of the time, why can't we get it right all of the time?

The discipline of quality improvement in healthcare is relatively young and this chapter explores its history and how thinking has emerged over time, together with the different aca-demic disciplines and the industries that improvement has drawn from. The field continues to evolve leading to a number of different approaches in contemporary practice.

Objectives

This chapter's objectives are to:

- Reflect on the history of quality in healthcare
- Discuss different approaches and models to improving quality in healthcare
- Describe the principles of quality improvement methodologies

A history of quality improvement

Hippocrates is generally considered to be the father of healthcare professions and is believed to have written an oath sometime between the fifth and third century B.C. In the oath, health-care professionals are required to declare that they will:

> devise and order for them [their patients] the best diet, according to my judgment and means; and I will take care that they suffer no hurt or damage.

> (Edelstein 1943)

This twin responsibility to both improve patients' health and avoid harm provides an ethi-cal base for clinical practice which is still relevant today. For most of history, the delivery of this promise has been seen to be the responsibility of individual practitioners, as suggested by Hippocrates, rather than of professional organisations or the state. The public safeguard was therefore to ensure that this clinical autonomy was only given to those in possession of expert knowledge and these practitioners then applied that knowledge as they judged best in local circumstances. Determining what constituted 'expert knowledge' became the responsibility of collectives who defined the standards of education and ethics and subsequently issued a licence for practice.

In the United Kingdom, the keepers of knowledge standards were at first the Guilds and then the Royal Colleges who guarded their own technical standards and controlled their use through supervised apprenticeships. As these organisations gained power, they were able to restrict work jurisdictions to those whom they had trained and to whom the organisation's membership had been granted. Maintenance of a continuing licence was dependent on adherence to collegiate standards and in return members were granted the privilege of autonomous practice. Quality was therefore assured by practitioners' admission and continued membership of the Guild or College.

The emergence of colleges for medical practitioners in the United Kingdom from the 1500s onwards and the granting of royal charters effectively restricted the practice of healthcare to their members. The definition of quality and agreement about what constituted appropriate interventions was made by these self-regulating colleges, albeit a number of competing colleges. Their claim of legitimate authority to set best practice standards went largely unchallenged, as other health workers had no similar accrediting college or guild, so the medical colleges increasingly set standards for the whole of the healthcare system.

Move to systems-based improvements

The focus on efficacy of the licenced practitioners' actions in relation to individual patients came under scrutiny with the scientific developments of the Enlightenment. The philosophical move from logical deduction to inductive reasoning through the collection of empirical data began to change the emphasis from the actions of individual practitioners to systems-based understanding of health. As early as 1546, Girolamo Fracastoro proposed that disease was transmitted through the air and therefore should be controlled by personal and environmental hygiene in addition to specific individual patient treatments (Nutton 1990). Developing this theme, in 1847, Ignaz Semmelweis collected data to understand why mortality rates differed between two different maternity clinics in one city. In an early example of using the study of variation to understand practice and reveal underlying factors that are not immediately apparent, Semmelweis collected empirical data that demonstrated that clinics run by medical practitioners and their students had higher death rates than those run by midwives and their students. Semmelweis proposed that medical staff were inadvertently cross infecting women following their anatomy dissection sessions. He introduced hand washing between cases which dramatically reduced mortality rates (see Box 1.1).

The central role of collecting data in understanding the causes of harm or quality failures was further demonstrated in 1854, when John Snow was able to demonstrate the importance of systems factors as well as individual patient factors when he methodically collected data about the location of the cholera cases (Shiode et al. 2015). Snow demonstrated that clusters of the disease were related to a contaminated water pump handle in Broad Street, London, and thus that environmental factors are as important as individual factors in improving health. Following quickly after this, Florence Nightingale (working with William Farr, Britain's foremost statistician at the time) was able to show that soldiers were 10 times more likely to die from infectious illnesses such as typhus, typhoid, cholera and dysentery than from wounds

Box 1.1 Case study: Reducing the incidence of puerperal fever in Vienna

In the early 1840s, the people of Vienna widely believed that there was a significant difference in death rates between two maternity clinics, although they did not understand why this should be. In a rare example of patient involvement in quality improvement, Semmelweis collected patient opinions and described desperate women begging not to be admitted to one of the clinics, preferring to deliver in the street without any professional assistance. Semmelweis's data suggested that even those who delivered without assistance had lower mortality rates than those who attended the other clinic, and he was puzzled that puerperal fever was rare among these women:

> To me, it appeared logical that patients who experienced street births would become ill at least as frequently as those who delivered in the clinic. . . . What protected those who delivered outside the clinic from these destructive unknown endemic influences?

By collecting data on all deaths, Semmelweis uncovered a significant variation with one clinic having a maternal mortality rate of 10%, whilst the other clinic had a mortality rate that was significantly less at 4%. Having uncovered the variation, Semmelweis began to look at what the differences in practice between the two clinics were. The only major difference that he could ascertain was that the clinic with high mortality rates was used as a teaching clinic for medical students, whilst the other had been used exclusively for training midwives since 1841.

His realisation of this distinction was important. Changes to medical training meant that dissection had become an important part of teaching medical students anatomy during the 1800s but was not a part of midwifery training. Semmelweis began to consider whether there was some process associated with dissection that was the cause of the variation. Semmelweis knew that a medical student had recently died following a needle stick injury during a dissection and that his post-mortem had shown similar pathology to that of the women who were dying from puerperal fever. Whilst the pathology techniques available at the time could not empirically identify the causal factor, Semmelweis hypothesised that the (unknown) causal agent was somehow being transmitted from the corpses being dissected to the labouring women.

Although Semmelweis did not understand how dissection and puerperal fever were linked, he noted that there was a putrid smell associated with infected autopsy tissue that was removed by hand washing. To test this logic, Semmelweis undertook a period of observation and noted that at the first clinic, doctors and medical students routinely moved from dissecting corpses to examining women without first washing their hands. He proposed that the practice of hand washing with chlorinated lime solutions destroyed the causal 'poisonous' or contaminating 'cadaveric' agent at the same time as removing the smell.

Semmelweis collected data before and after his improvement and showed dramatic reductions in mortality after hand washing was introduced, with maternal mortality at the first clinic dropping from 10% to 1%.

(Continued)

Box 1.1 Case study: Reducing the incidence of puerperal fever in Vienna (*Continued*)

Despite very clear data to support his improvement, Semmelweis's observations conflicted with the established scientific and medical opinions of the time, and his ideas were rejected by the medical community. Semmelweis thus encountered the problem that persists today – evidence alone is not sufficient to sustain and spread even dramatic quality improvements.

Source: Semmelweis, I. *The Cause, Concept, and Prophylaxis of Childbed Fever* (translated by Carter, K., 1983), University of Wisconsin Press, London, 1861.

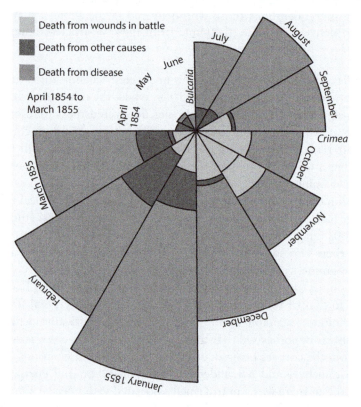

Figure 1.1 A coxcomb chart displaying causes of mortality among soldiers in the Crimea. (From Nightingale, F., *Notes on Matters Affecting the Health, Efficiency, and Hospital Administration of the British Army: Founded Chiefly on the Experience of the Late War*, Presented by Request to the Secretary of State for War, Harrison and Sons London, 1858.)

acquired in battle (Nightingale 1858). Her creative use of data visualisation such as her coxcomb charts (see Figure 1.1) persuaded politicians to send the Sanitary Commission to the Crimea in March 1855. The resulting flushing of the sewers and improvement in the ventilation resulted in a sharp reduction in mortality rates. Florence Nightingale was honoured for her applied use of statistics by becoming the first woman elected to become a member of the Royal Statistical Society in 1858.

Using data for quality control

Advances in the use of data to explore the causes of adverse events led to increasing ınıcı_. in its use to measure the degree of control of quality of healthcare processes. Previously, the state had played no role in defining the competency of healthcare practitioners, but the emergence of tools to assess the quality of care (or more precisely, its absence) and the growth of empirical research or 'evidence' for interventions led to the statutory regulation of healthcare practitioners (as opposed to the voluntary registration with professional colleges), making it illegal to practise without having demonstrated achievement of national standards of education and competence.

The Medical Act of 1858, an Act of the United Kingdom Parliament, created (for the first time in the world) a register of 'qualified' medical practitioners. This was followed by the creation of statutory registers in the United Kingdom for midwives in 1902, nurses in 1919 (despite vigorous opposition from Florence Nightingale) and dentists in 1948. Currently, internationally most health professions are either subject to statutory registration or professional accreditation, indeed in some cases, a combination of the two. In recent years, the dynamic aspect of practice has been recognised, and there has been a move from single point licensing to periodic revalidation which requires demonstration of ongoing competence. This was introduced in the United Kingdom for medical practitioners in 2012 and for nurses and midwives in 2016.

Clinical audit

The move to statutory registration was followed by a move to using data to assure compliance with professional standards through the process of audit. In 1912, Ernest Codman asserted that every patient should be followed up after surgery to identify what he called 'the end results', which would now be called outcomes (Neuhauser 1990). He went on to establish the American College of Surgeons' systematic study of the outcomes for all the individual patients of each surgeon leading to the establishment of their Hospital Standardization Program in 1917 with five common standards for all hospitals.

Codman's 'end results' approach was further developed during the 1960s by Avis Donabedian, who proposed a broader definition of quality, noting the interdependence of outcomes with both structures and processes (Donabedian 1989). Donabedian's model recognises that the actions of individuals and groups of practitioners (processes) combine with the context and resources available to create the outcomes and that exploring either structure or process alone would not improve care. The introduction of evidence-based medicine (Cochrane 1972) to research and disseminating the evidence of what works accelerated the use of audit, initially focused on patient outcome as a way of examining the practice of individuals, and then later, the practice of teams.

Following regional examples, the United Kingdom formalised the audits of deaths through the National Confidential Enquiry into Maternal Deaths in 1952, and this was followed by the National Confidential Enquiry into Patient Outcome and Death in 1988. In 1989, the UK National Health Service (NHS) was formally required by government to undertake medical audit, which was defined as:

> The systematic critical analysis of the quality of medical care including the procedures used for diagnosis and treatment, the use of resources and the resulting outcome and quality of life for the patient.

(Department of Health [DH] 1989)

Very soon afterwards, audit requirements were extended beyond medicine to include all healthcare professions and renamed clinical audit. In the United Kingdom, there are currently a number of national audit programmes and also peer review programmes, such as the cancer peer review networks, which are complemented by many thousands of local team audits that provide a lens to the quality of services.

Accreditation

Codman's hospital standards audit gained traction, and by 1952 a number of different medical colleges in the United States came together to form the Joint Commission on Accreditation of Hospitals, a voluntary scheme which currently accredits more than 21,000 healthcare organisations in the United States. The success of the Joint Commission was a trigger to the American Nurses' Association, which created the American Nurses' Credentialing Centre to offer the Magnet Hospital Recognition Program for Excellence in Nursing Services.

Accreditation is based on the assumption that adhering to standards will produce higher quality services and an increasingly safe environment. The accreditation model has spread across the world and is now an integral part of quality assurance in over 70 countries. Pomey et al. (2005) raised the question about whether accreditation differs from inspection and suggested that this depends on the extent to which it is voluntary or mandatory and linked to legislation and sanction. Whilst a number of countries, for example France, have instigated a mandatory accreditation scheme, the United Kingdom has instead relied on internal review and in 1999 required all providers of services to the NHS to introduce a governance system for clinical care. Clinical Governance was defined as:

> A system through which NHS organisations are accountable for continually improving the quality of their services and safeguarding high standards of care by creating an environment in which clinical care will flourish.
>
> (Scally and Donaldson 1998, p. 62)

Clinical Governance comprised the following seven 'pillars':

- Audit
- Clinical effectiveness
- Risk management
- Patient involvement
- Use of information
- Education and training
- Staffing and management

These pillars reflect the domains of accreditation and inspection found in other countries and focus on self-management of compliance with standards and the collection of evidence. The NHS provider organisations were given a statutory responsibility for the quality of care (previously this had lain with individual clinical professionals), marking a sea of change and a move towards corporate accountability.

Accreditation assumes that compliance with standards will improve quality but is not explicit about the mechanism by which this happens. Compliance and improvement are not synonymous, and whilst meeting standards is important, Pomey et al. (2005) suggested that improvement can only happen:

If there are 'spaces of freedom' for the professionals and positive incentive mechanisms for its realization. (p. 53)

Accreditation and inspection might be useful, even necessary, but moving from awareness of performance to improvement requires further action.

From quality control to quality improvement

In 1913, Henry Ford began an experiment. His company had been building cars one at a time but this was time consuming and therefore expensive. In his search for a more efficient process, Ford broke down the components of the system and developed machines that could make individual components separately from each other. He then successfully introduced the idea of building a linear process with a sequential set of tasks which could be undertaken by unskilled workers to assemble these parts into a complete car. This method evolved into his highly successful car manufacturing production line, which was able to produce a high volume of parts that were later combined to produce low-cost cars. Ford's production line was revolutionary and quickly became the benchmark for mass production across the world.

Quality in the production line was managed by inspecting and controlling which finished products got into the supply chain. Quality control meant that the customer did not receive faulty parts but did nothing to eliminate the faulty parts. Whilst the low cost of the production of the parts enabled his company to flourish, the existence of defective parts was considered to be the price paid for quality. This approach dominated manufacturing for most of the twentieth century with targets and thresholds for quality failure being the main device to improve the product, without necessarily addressing the defective parts. However, this acceptance of an element of quality failure was challenged as early as 1918 by Walter Shewhart.

Shewhart worked at the Western Electric Company Inspection Engineering Department at the Hawthorne Works where a number of experiments were undertaken to explore how productivity and quality could be increased (including the famous experiment that bears the Hawthorne name, which showed that any change in work conditions increased productivity for a short time). Shewhart (1939) proposed that quality is better achieved by the prevention of defective outputs rather than inspecting them out of the supply; or to put it another way, it is better to get it right first time. Using statistical tests, he observed significant variations within the same process over time and concluded that the quality could be improved through reducing variation in a process to produce a more consistent and reliable product. Reducing variations would also reduce the waste associated with the quality control where defective products or process failures are tolerated and managed out of the systems rather than eliminated.

Shewhart also observed that variation within a process follows two distinct patterns in the data, suggesting that there are two distinct types of variation which he proposed should each be managed in a different way. Some variation is related to the process design but remains within limits predicted from past performance, and Shewhart called this 'common cause variation'. When variation is outside these predicted limits, he claimed this is related to external factors and called this special cause variation. Improving a process will not reduce variation caused by factors that are outside the design, and so it is important to understand the type of variation to determine the management action.

Shewhart devised a visual representation of variation over time to monitor the reliability of a process. Statistical process control (SPC) charts (see Chapter 6) use continuous data to plot the extent and type of variation. The range of common cause variation (related to the design of the process) can be calculated by determining plus or minus three standard deviations (if the data has a normal distribution) of variation over time. When the subsequent variation falls within the predicted limits, the system is said to be within statistical control, and therefore the quality is determined entirely by the process itself. The aim of quality improvement is then to make the process more reliable by reducing the range of variation which will be reflected by reducing the distance between the control limits. Data outside the predicted control limits indicates that factors outside the current process are influencing the measure, and these external factors need further investigation; if they occur regularly, then a redesign of the process might be needed. Shewhart was successful in increasing the reliability of processes through both reducing the range of variation and redesigning process and therefore reducing the waste which is a byproduct of quality control systems.

In 1925, Shewhart moved to the Bell Telephone Laboratories and continued his work on improvement process quality. There he continued the development of his statistical approaches and started a long collaboration with W. Edwards Deming. Shewhart's charts were adopted by the American Society for Testing Materials (ASTM) in 1933, and both Shewhart and Deming were employed to work on improving production of materials for the United States during the Second World War.

Deming's profound knowledge

After the war, the United States led the efforts of the Allies to rebuild the Japanese state, including sending experts to Japan to help rebuild the economy. One of those experts was Deming, who introduced Shewhart's theories to manufacturing industries, particularly Toyota. Whilst Deming remained convinced of the importance of measuring variation, he became increasingly aware of the need to set that within a wider context. Deming's work at Toyota heavily influenced his thinking, and he noted 'knowing the numbers doesn't give you the answers, only the questions that need to be asked' (Gabor 1990, p. 126). Deming cautioned that information should not be confused with knowledge and that information without rigorous application of theory does not produce knowledge or improvement. His work in Japan led him to describe four principles of a quality improvement paradigm that form a conceptual framework for quality improvement, which he called profound knowledge (see Box 1.2).

Deming's first principle of profound knowledge is the appreciation of a system. He emphasised the interconnectedness of the different components of a system and that reducing a process to a set of independent tasks without an understanding of the whole system, and the role that each part being studied plays within the system, risked improvement activities at best failing and at worst causing unintended consequences elsewhere in the system. Deming asserted that making the whole system work requires coordination and cooperation of the parts, and this is achieved through leadership. The system leader must

---

Box 1.2 Profound knowledge: Deming's (1986) four principles

1   Appreciation of a system
2   Understanding the theory of knowledge
3   Psychology of change
4   Knowledge about variation

ensure that there is a shared understanding and commitment to the common purpose of the system before improvement on one element can be successfully achieved. It is therefore important that an improvement activity, even if a small project limited to one part of it, is considered within the system context and that the improvement project is coordinated through the system leader.

Deming's second principle is an understanding of the theory of knowledge. Knowledge is developed from the application of theory and creating and testing hypotheses from the available evidence. He cautions that it is then important to be sure that there is deep understanding of theory because, he asserts, improvement is an iterative process that is driven by a theory that leads to predictions (hypotheses), which are then tested and measured empirically. Understanding the theoretical mechanism by which improvement happens is necessary in order that the data required to measure whether the process worked as intended can be identified. Improvement activities must therefore be based on a clear, evidence-based theory that leads to a hypothesis that is then tested in practice.

Deming's third principle addresses the psychology of change. Improvement is a form of change and requires the support of the individuals involved in the process. Deming believed that people could not be instructed to change their behaviours but should be motivated to change through a sense of shared purpose and alignment of the improvement interventions with existing work processes. The shared purpose may be actively developed, facilitated by the leadership, or it may develop organically, but it is this motivation that determines whether the evidence-based intervention is adopted.

Deming's fourth principle, knowledge about variation, reflects Shewhart's seminal work on the need to understand the cause of variation. Deming believed that individuals are limited by the design of a process and that knowledge of variation is primarily a diagnostic tool about the process. Using a single, post-intervention outcome measure does not reveal anything about the process design. If the single measure shows improvement, the goodness of the process is not questioned, but if the next point gets worse, the process may be assumed to have failed, when in fact both may reflect the common cause variation resulting from the same process. Knowing the range of variation is far more effective for evaluating the quality than making a judgement from a single data point.

Deming described how the principles of profound knowledge are used in practice to improve quality through the Shewhart Plan, Do, Check, Act (PDCA) cycle (Dale 2003) of continuous improvement consisting of:

- Planning based on external evidence and internal performance data that are used to predict how an intervention will make an improvement
- Doing the implementation, using the psychology of change
- Checking resulting effects on the system, whether the desired results occur
- Taking action to fully implement the changes or plan a new intervention

The plan is based on knowledge (from theory) that leads to a hypothesis of what will bring about improvement in a given situation. This is then tested in the 'do' phase. The consequences or outcomes of the action (the doing) are checked for variation leading to action that refines the theory and improves the intervention.

The cycle is repeated in an iterative manner to achieve continuous rather than episodic improvement as the checking of the testing (doing) phase leads to further refinement of the theory, and new hypotheses are generated and tested. In this way, quality is continuously improved. Later in his career, Deming (1993) changed the cycle name from PDCA to Plan, Do, Study, Act (PDSA) as he felt that some people were interpreting the C (checking), as measuring compliance with the intervention (a throwback to quality control systems), rather than analysis of the impact of the intervention and looking at how it could be improved, which he described as 'studying'. It is the evaluative nature of the PDSA that makes quality improvement a continuous rather than a control process, and it might therefore properly be called a spiral rather than a cycle.

From PDSA to LEAN

Deming's work in Japan was highly successful and was adopted and further developed into the Toyota Production System which emphasised the elimination of waste that can be a byproduct of quality control systems. The term 'LEAN was coined by Womack and Jones (1996) during the late 1980s to describe Toyota's approach and is described more as a philosophy than a methodology. Womack and Jones articulated five principles of LEAN (see Box 1.3). Chapter 3 addresses LEAN in more detail.

The real achievement of the Toyota Production System is described by Spear (2004) as not merely the creation and use of the tools they developed, but the fact that it created a culture in which all work is seen as a series of nested, ongoing experiments, embedding quality improvement in the everyday work of all the employees, not just a specific department or isolated project. This sort of systems thinking is also the basis of recent emphasis on organisational learning (Senge 1990). It can be described as exploration of 'the properties which exist once the parts (of the system) have been combined into a whole' (Iles and Sutherland 2001, p. 17).

Other schools of quality improvement

A number of different schools of quality improvement emerged in Japan, including Six Sigma, Total Quality Management (TQM) and Quality Circles. The 'golden thread' through all of them is that improvement, as opposed to simply control, is fundamental to quality and therefore must permeate the culture of the whole organisation rather than be in the hands of a single department.

Whilst quality improvement approaches were paying dividends in Japan, they were less well known in English speaking countries which were still relying on quality control until the economic crises of the 1970s and 1980s led business leaders to explore ways of ensuring quality at a lower cost. In 1982, Peters and Waterman published their book, In Search of Excellence, which suggested that the Japanese whole system approaches to quality were

---

Box 1.3 Principles of LEAN

- Identification of what constitutes value to the client.
- Management of the value stream, that is, the activities that create value.
- Developing the capability to ensure that the different parts of the production system flow.
- Use of 'pull' mechanisms to flow, the 'just in time' principle.
- The pursuit of perfection through reducing all forms of waste in the system.

Source: Womack, J. and Jones, D., *Lean Thinking: Banish Waste and Create Wealth in Your Organisation*, Simon & Shuster, New York, NY, 1996.

the key to excellence and cost efficiency. This triggered interest in how the systems-based approaches to quality could be applied across a range of industries.

Systems thinking in healthcare

The well known aphorism that every system is perfectly designed to achieve the results it achieves has a corollary that changing the results must require a change in the system. Following Peters and Waterman's (1982) call for systems-based quality management for business, healthcare systems around the world started to explore how this might work for them. There was renewed interest in Donabedian's model, with its inclusion of structural and process elements that began to explore how context and resources, as well as the actions of individuals, contribute to patient outcomes. This model was used, for example, by the United Kingdom's Royal College of Nursing (RCN) in 1985 to develop its dynamic standard setting system (DySSSy). The RCN shifted the focus of audit from national guidelines, asserting that it should be locally designed by those who give care, thus encouraging nurses and other health professionals to take ownership of quality and set standards in the context of their own local work settings.

The UK Department of Health's 1989 white paper *Working for Patients* challenged the role of the professional in assuring their own practice, and the government funded 23 TQM pilots based on Japanese quality management principles. Reviewing TQM in the NHS, Berwick (1992a) suggested that the principles of TQM offered promise and that 'with appropriate modifications, these principles can apply to the work of medicine' (p. 304).

At the same time as continuous improvement was being explored in the United Kingdom, in the United States, the National Demonstration Project on Quality Improvement in Health Care began to look for new approaches to quality in healthcare, largely because of their perceived local failures to act on the results of audit to achieve meaningful change (Berwick et al. 1992b). Berwick's work led to the establishment in 1991 of the Institute of Healthcare Improvement (IHI), whose mission was to redesign healthcare into a system without errors, waste, delay and unsustainable costs. In 1996, the IHI adopted the Associates in Process Improvement (API) Model for Improvement (Langley et al. 1996) for its Breakthrough Series Collaborative. The Model for Improvement drew heavily on Deming and Shewhart's work and advocated the use of PDSA cycles with the addition of three questions to articulate Deming's Theory of Knowledge, which are as follows:

1 What are we trying to achieve?
2 How will we know that a change is an improvement?
3 What changes can we make that will result in improvement?

See Figure 1.2 for the model of improvement (Langley et al. 2009).

The IHI emphasises the use of measurement plans and recommends starting immediately with tests of changes on a small scale over a short period and refining the intervention until the desired outcome is achieved. Once the aim is successfully achieved, the testing is broadened and the improvement project scaled up to other areas. The IHI Breakthrough Series was an exploration of how improvement could be achieved at scale. It began with a project to reduce caesarean rates, first at a local then a regional and then a national (U.S.) level. The IHI quickly began to use the model internationally, starting in Sweden and Norway in 1997 and Holland and the United Kingdom in 1999. The extent to which the model has achieved its aim of sustained, large-scale improvement, however, remains uncertain.

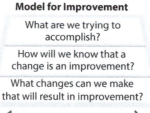

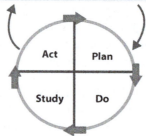

Figure 1.2 Model for improvement. (Langley et al. *The Improvement Guide.* 2009. Copyright Wiley-VCH Verlag GmbH & Co. KGaA. Reproduced with permission.*)*

The pace of application of different quality improvement methods accelerated following a number of key reports that illustrated the extent to which systems failure causes harm to patients. The Institute of Medicine's (IOM) report 'To Err is Human' (Kohn et al. 1999) published with the startling claim that in the United States between 44,000 and 98,000 people die each year as a result of preventable healthcare errors. This was followed in the United Kingdom by the Chief Medical Officer's report 'Organisation with a memory' in 2000 (Donaldson 2000) which echoed the IOM findings by reporting that 1 in 10 people admitted to the NHS experienced an adverse event related to their healthcare. These shocking figures reflected the realisation that harm is not always a result of incompetence or negligence but could also be due to the way individuals interact with the system.

Reason (2000) differentiated between active failures (actions or omissions by individuals) and latent failures (the context that allows the actions) using the analogy of mosquitoes:

> Active failures are like mosquitoes. They can be swatted one by one, but they still keep coming. The best remedies are to create more effective defences and to drain the swamps in which they breed. The swamps, in this case, are the ever present latent conditions. (p. 769)

Thus, quality failures occur when the nature of the task, the organisational conditions and the human factors come together to create a perfect storm. Reason (2000) described this as being similar to Swiss cheese, providing an illustration of where the holes in Swiss cheese line up together by chance.

Human factors

The move toward systems thinking has been criticised by some who caution against ignoring the agency or action of humans within the system and assert that systems are only as effective as the people who work within them. Quality improvement therefore requires a consideration of how people interact with each other and the system. This reflects both Deming's focus on the psychology of change and Donabedian's recognition of the balance of structure and agency, and recent developments in quality improvement thinking have increasingly sought to integrate human factors into improvement methodologies.

Human factors are defined as:

> Environmental, organisational and job factors, and human and individual characteristics which influence behaviour at work in a way which can affect health and safety. (Health and Safety Executive 1999, p. 2)

A scientific discipline has emerged that applies theory, principles, data and methods to design in order to optimise human well-being and overall system performance, drawing on a number of academic traditions. Psychologists, including James Reason and Charles Vincent, have led much of the application of human factors theory to patient safety in healthcare.

Human factors theory recognises that humans are both risks and assets to healthcare systems. Humans can respond in an agile way to the unexpected, but their performance can also be influenced in an unhelpful way in unexpected or imperfect conditions. Humans cannot be redesigned, and so the management of latent conditions, rather than the training of people, is seen to be the best way of strengthening defences and barriers. This involves designing systems that make it difficult for people to take the wrong actions, prompt them to take desired actions and introduce processes to ensure that lapses and errors are identified and acted upon without becoming system failures. An example of this is the standardisation of infusion pumps to avoid errors in programming flow rates when a member of staff under pressure assumes the operation is the same for pumps made by different manufacturers or the introduction of different tips on syringes to ensure that preparations for oral use are not inadvertently administrated via the parenteral route.

Another example of human factors is the need for clear and effective communication of key information. Situation, Background, Assessment, Recommendation (SBAR) is a pro forma for communication in critical situations developed by the U.S. military to provide a standardised, predictable structure to the message, and SBAR has been successfully applied in healthcare (Haig et al. 2006). The common structure means both the person making the communication and the person receiving it have a shared expectation of what needs to be included, and there is therefore a double check that all critical information has been shared.

Exploring how system design can guide humans and increase their situational awareness can enhance the more traditional approaches to quality improvement by increasing the capacity to address unexpected or unusual circumstances. As quality improvement projects move into more and more complex and unpredictable scenarios, there is increasing interest in the concept of quality as reliability.

High Reliability Organisations

Despite increasing attention to the evidence base for healthcare interventions, it is clear that implementing the recommendations is highly context specific. In a landmark study in 2003, McGlynn et al. telephoned a random sample of adults living in 12 metropolitan areas in the United States and asked them about their healthcare experiences. They also reviewed their healthcare records for the previous 2-year period to discern their status in relation to 439 indicators of quality of care across 30 diagnostic conditions. They found that only 54.9% of the adults they were studying had received the gold standard of recommended care. A similar study in the United Kingdom (Burnett et al. 2012) examined the reliability of the following four clinical processes in the NHS:

1   Handover between staff for medical in-patients
2   Prescribing against formulary
3   Availability of clinical notes and results
4   Cross-organisational communication for care of older people

Burnett et al. concluded that there was a failure to meet the agreed standards between 13% and 19% of the time, meaning that up to one in five patients were not receiving the best quality care. This increasing attention on reliability reflects Shewhart's work on the range of variation within a system that is in overall control and that averages conceal inconsistent practice and experiences.

Reliability is not the same as standardisation; it is described as 'the lack of unwanted, unanticipated, and unexplainable variance in performance' (Hollnagel 1993, p. 51). In predictable and stable and closed systems, where there is little reason to vary, this may be interpreted as standardising actions and processes and demanding complete compliance with them. This can be highly effective in the appropriate circumstances; however, it can also be highly dangerous in less certain conditions. Standardisation cannot accommodate the unexpected as Weick et al. (2008) found:

> The singular focus on repeatability as the primary defining quality of reliability in traditional definitions, fails to deal with the reality that reliable systems often must perform the same way even though their working conditions fluctuate and are not always known in advance. For a system to remain reliable, it must somehow handle unforeseen situations in ways that forestall unintended consequences. (p. 36)

Variation is inherent in healthcare because of the unpredictability of the patient flow, the individuality of the patients and the number of different members of staff delivering care to the same patient (Haraden and Resar 2004). This unpredictability cannot be eliminated, and so quality systems based on standardisation are likely to have only partial success, thus leading many healthcare improvers to start looking at how other industries with unstable conditions manage quality.

Studies of industries that have a high risk of the unexpected but also have low rates of quality failure have identified the concept of High Risk Organisations (HROs), which operate in complex, dynamic environments where there is constant risk of unpredictable events. Despite being in very different industries, HROs share a number of common features. They all perform reliably, despite the changing circumstances, through their focus on predicting, detecting, containing and bouncing back from variation in conditions.

HROs recognise that whilst organisational variability is one of the greatest risks, it is also one of an organisation's greatest strengths. Whilst systems are designed to follow best practice for what is anticipated, the ability to identify the unexpected and vary actions as appropriate is what maintains the reliability and therefore quality. In predictable situations, HROs follow the same processes as many other organisations and have default protocols; what singles them out is their ability to detect the unexpected and immediately switch from protocol-driven practice to local expertise and to then revert back to the routine process once the unexpected has been mitigated. A prime example of HRO working is the armed forces. Military organisations work in very hierarchical teams with strong accountability and clear unambiguous procedures during routine work but revert to local command during combat.

In order to operate two apparently divergent management systems, HROs have developed a set of shared goals and established consistent assumptions that drive the local expertise. This illustrates how HROs are dependent on collective mindfulness; that is a shared understanding of real-time operations in order to anticipate changes and seamlessly switch their thinking in order to contain unwanted variation.

Weick et al.'s (2008) study of High Reliability Organisations describes two key factors that set them apart from less reliable counterparts: anticipation and containment. Anticipation is achieved through three components. First a preoccupation with failure, accepting that not everything can be controlled and that the unexpected will happen. By accepting the inevitability of the unexpected, HROs constantly look for what might cause process failure. This mindfulness means that they avoid the 'arrogance of optimism' and scan for early warnings of it. Anticipating failure also leads HROs to have well developed plans to mitigate it. Second, there is a reluctance to simplify and an understanding that in the real world things are not linear and do not progress in a chronological order so reducing data to averages and targets can give a false sense of security. Third, there is an acute sensitivity to operations; instead of managing through the use of historical data, reflecting Deming's television comments in 1980 that 'management by results is like driving a car by looking in the rear view mirror', HROs monitor as much as possible in real time, thus picking up patterns that give early warnings of deviations and therefore potential to prevent them from increasing. These three components create a shared understanding across all the staff that Weick et al. describe as 'collective mindfulness'.

Weick et al. (2008) observed that once a potential failure has been identified, it needs to be contained. HROs are able to contain it through two routes. First they have developed personal and organisational resilience through creating a culture in which the organisation can cope with uncertainty and has the ability to implement back up plans. An important feature of HROs is their collective preparedness. They expect to make errors and train their workforce to recognise and recover them rather than blame them. HROs view untoward events as a valuable resource from which they can learn and build the organisational resilience. Second, they ensure expertise is constantly available at the frontline (rather than through remote supervision), which allows them to rapidly move from protocol driven activity to context-specific decisions based on the local expertise.

Quality is therefore defined not as preventing isolated failures, either human or technical or by meeting specific targets or metrics, but as the degree of capacity to calibrate actions to maintain reliable performance. HROs do this by making the system as robust as is practicable in the face of its human and operational hazards so that continuity and reliability of the system is maintained.

Patient involvement

The most recent and still emergent approach to quality improvement in healthcare is patient and public engagement; this will be addressed in detail in Chapter 4. The scope of lay involvement in improvement is contested and there are a number of different discourses being played out. Justifications for involving patients in improvement projects are broadly similar to those for lay involvement in healthcare more generally. For some, it is solely about the patient experience whilst for others it is about framing patients and the public as funders who therefore have a legitimate stake in designing health services. As Harry Cayton observed, it is all too easy to collapse all aspects of patient and public involvement into a 'single portmanteau concept', which may not be particularly helpful (House of Commons Select Committee on Health 2007, p. 10).

Conclusion

Assessing and improving the quality of healthcare services has always been important but the mechanisms to attempt to achieve this have changed through history, leading to a vigorous debate about whether quality improvement and increasingly patient safety in healthcare should constitute a new field for health services research (Grol and Wensing 2004).

Some have deemed 'improvement science' as a new academic discipline whilst others suggest it is the application of existing health systems research, health and behavioural economics, epidemiology, statistics, organisation and management science and sociology. What is increasingly clear is that knowing what should be done is not enough. Knowing how to make it happen consistently, in different circumstances and across a large system is challenging and requires a great deal of consideration.

From a starting point of reliance on the competence of individuals through quality control systems, there is currently increasing interest on the impact of context and culture on quality improvement and some doubt whether there can ever be an 'optimal methodology' (Grol and Wensing 2004). It is therefore important for healthcare improvers to develop a working knowledge of a range of concepts and methods and to constantly improve their own knowledge and skill in applying it.

References

Associates in Process Improvement (n.d.) *Associates in Process Improvement Model of Improvement.* Available from: http://www.apiweb.org/ (accessed on 8 July 2016).

Berwick, D., Enthoven, A., and Bunker, J. (1992a) Quality management in the NHS: The doctor's role – II. *British Medical Journal* 304: 304–308.

Berwick, D., Enthoven, A., and Bunker J. (1992b) Quality management in the NHS: The actions of formal and informal leaders. In the doctor's role – I. *British Medical Journal* 304: 235–239.

Burnett, S., Franklin, B.D., Moorthy, K., Cooke, M.W., and Vincent, C. (2012) How reliable are clinical systems in the UK NHS? A study of seven NHS organisations. *British Medical Journal Quality and Safety* 21(6): 466–472.

Cochrane, A. (1972) *Effectiveness and Efficiency: Random Reflections on Health Services.* London: Nuffield Provincial Hospitals Trust.

Dale, B., editor (2003) *Managing Quality.* Oxford: Blackwell Publishing.

Deming, W. (1986) *Out of the Crisis.* Cambridge, MA: MIT Center for Advanced Engineering Study.

Deming, W.E. (1993) *The New Economics.* Cambridge, MA: MIT Press. Department of Health. (1989) *Working for Patients.* Working paper No. 6. London: HMSO.

Donabedian, A. (1989) The end results of health care: Ernest Codman's contribution to quality assessment and beyond. *Milbank Quarterly* 67(2): 233–256.

Donaldson, L. (2000) *An Organisation with a Memory: Report of an Expert Group on Learning from Adverse Events in the NHS.* Norwich: Stationery Office.

Edelstein, L. (1943) *The Hippocratic Oath: Text, Translation and Interpretation.* Baltimore, MD: Johns Hopkins Press.

Ford Company (n.d.) *The Evolution of Mass Production.* Available from: http://www.ford.co.uk/experience-ford/Heritage/EvolutionOfMassProduction (accessed on 8 July 2016).

Gabor, A. (1990) *The Man Who Discovered Quality: How W. Edwards Deming Brought the Quality Revolution to America.* New York, NY: Penguin Books.

Grol, R. and Wensing, M. (2004) What drives change? Barriers to and incentives for achieving evidence-based practice. *Medical Journal of Australia* 180(6): S57.

Health and Safety Executive (1999) *Reducing Error and Influencing Behaviour.* HSG 48. London: HMSO.

Haig, K.M., Sutton, S., and Whittington, J. (2006) SBAR: A shared mental model for improving communication between clinicians. *The Joint Commission Journal on Quality and Patient Safety* 32(3): 167–175.

Haraden, C. and Resar, R. (2004) Patient flow in hospitals: Understanding and controlling it better. *Frontiers of Health Services Management* 20(4): 3–15.

Hollnagel, E. (1993) *Human Reliability Analysis: Context and Control*. London: Academic Press.

House of Commons Select Committee on Health (2007) *Patient and Public Involvement in the NHS*. Third Report of Session 2006–07, Vol. 1. London: HMSO.

Iles, V. and Sutherland, K. (2001) *Managing Change in the NHS. Organisational Change: A Review for Health Care Managers, Professionals, and Researchers*. London: NCCSDO.

Kohn, L., Corrigan, J., and Donaldson, M. (1999) *To Err is Human. Building a Safer Health System. Committee on Quality of Health Care in America*. Washington, DC: Institute of Medicine.

Langley,H., Moen, R., Nolan, K., Nolan, T., Norman, C., and Provost, L. (2009) *The Improvement Guide*. 2nd Edition. San Francisco, CA: Jossey-Bass.

Langley, G., Nolan, K., Nolan, K., Norman, C., and Provost, L. (1996) *The Improvement Guide: A Practical Guide to Enhancing Organizational Performance*. San Francisco, CA: Jossey-Bass.

McGlynn, E.A., Asch, S.M., Adams, J., Keesey, J., Hicks, J., DeCristofaro, A., and Kerr, E.A. (2003) The quality of health care delivered to adults in the United States. *New England Journal of Medicine* 348(26): 2635–2645.

Neuhauser, D. (1990) Ernest Amory Codman, MD, and end results of medical care. *International Journal of Technology Assessment in Health Care* 6(2): 307–325.

Nightingale, F. (1858) *Notes on Matters Affecting the Health, Efficiency, and Hospital Administration of the British Army: Founded Chiefly on the Experience of the Late War*. Presented by Request to the Secretary of State for War. London: Harrison and Sons.

Nutton, V. (1990) The reception of fracastoro's theory of contagion: The seed that fell among thorns? *Osiris* 6: 196–234.

Peters, T. and Waterman, R. (1982) *In Search of Excellence: Lessons from America's Best-Run Companies*. New York, NY: Harper & Row.

Pomey, M., Francois, P., Contandriopoulos, A., Tosh, A., and Bertrand, D. (2005) Paradoxes of French accreditation. *Quality and Safety in Health Care* 14(1): 51–55.

Reason, J. (2000) Human error: Models and management. *British Medical Journal* 320(7237): 768–770.

Scally, G. and Donaldson, L.J. (1998) Clinical governance and the drive for QI in the new NHS in England. *British Medical Journal* 317: 61–65.

Semmelweis, I. (1861) *The Cause, Concept, and Prophylaxis of Childbed Fever* (translated by Carter, K., 1983), Vol. 2. London: University of Wisconsin Press.

Senge, P. (1990) *The Fifth Discipline: The Art and Science of the Learning Organization*. New York, NY: Currency Doubleday.

Shiode, N., Shiode, S., Rod-Thatcher, E., Rana, S., and Vinten-Johansen, P. (2015) The mortality rates and the space-time patterns of John Snow's cholera epidemic map. *International Journal of Health Geographics* 14(1): 21–36.

Spear, S. (2004) Learning to lead at Toyota. *Harvard Business Review* 82(5): 78–91.

Shewhart, W. (1939) *Statistical Method from the Viewpoint of Quality Control*. Washington, DC: The Graduate School of the Department of Agriculture.

Weick, K., Sutcliffe, K., and Obstfeld, D. (2008) Organizing for high reliability: Processes of collective mindfulness. *Crisis Management* 3(1): 81–123.

Womack, J. and Jones, D. (1996) *Lean Thinking: Banish Waste and Create Wealth in Your Organisation*. New York, NY: Simon & Shuster.

2 Understanding the Context for Healthcare Improvement

Elaine Maxwell and Lesley Baillie

Introduction

Context is a major influencing factor for the translation of quality improvement theory into practice in healthcare (Leslie et al. 2014), and so understanding context, including climate and culture, is important for improvement work (Kirchner et al. 2012). Healthcare organisations operate in environments 'characterised as resource-constrained, time pressured and highly political' (Greenfield et al. 2011, p. 336). The complexity and multifaceted nature of healthcare systems cannot be overemphasised (Kirchner et al. 2012) within such a context, and implementing improvement requires understanding of the social impact of changes and of the strategies that engage staff within organisations (Greenfield et al. 2011).

This chapter introduces context and explores the influences on improvement of the content of the change proposed, the context for improvement and the processes undertaken during improvement. The nature of culture and climate and their effects on improvement are also examined, with ethnography explored as a way of understanding context. Organisational readiness for change and ways of assessing readiness are considered, and we include examples of how contextual factors affect quality improvements to illuminate these concepts.

Objectives

The chapter's objectives are to:

- Examine theories and models that explain context in relation to organisational readiness and the variation of improvement success in practice
- Analyse the content-context process model in relation to healthcare improvement
- Consider tools for assessment of organisational readiness for change
- Reflect on how organisational culture and climate relate to the context for healthcare improvement
- Explore ethnography as a way of understanding the organisational culture and context for healthcare improvement

Introducing context

The advent of the Internet has led to an explosion in the availability of the evidence base for healthcare. The clinical evidence base has been used in many quality improvement programmes to create structured process pathways that should lead to reliably good patient outcomes, and yet considerable variation occurs even in the most clearly defined care delivery systems. Repeated studies have shown that planned change has, at best, a 30% chance of sustained change (Øvretveit et al. 2002; Self and Schraeder 2009).

Evidence is collected largely through research in which the context is controlled; hence the predominant view that the gold standard for evidence is randomised controlled trials (RCTs). Large amounts of data are analysed to produce statistical generalisations about the probability of a cause and effect. Whilst this gives incredibly helpful detail of what might be expected to happen in ideal circumstances, the evidence needs to be considered in the light of the fact that local practice contexts very rarely match idealised research contexts and indeed can differ significantly from one unit to the next or even one time frame to another. When seeking the best improvement design for a specific improvement project, it is important to understand and embrace the variations in context and this must begin with its assessment.

The importance of understanding context was well demonstrated by the increasing interest in the reasons for the competitive advantage of Japanese manufacturers over the United States during the 1960s and 1970s. Review of the Japanese success led Peters and Waterman (1982) to reject the view that change could be managed through a standardised, centralised plan, and they proposed that understanding the context, and in particular the organisational culture, is key to improvement. Their book, *In Search of Excellence*, reflected seismic changes in the way U.S. industry started to look at improvement and the growing interest in what else, other than the innovation, would be important to determining success. Thirty years later, Kaplan et al. (2010) conducted a systematic review of literature to identify contextual factors that affected success of quality improvement initiatives within healthcare. They defined context as anything not directly part of the technical quality improvement process and the clinical interventions. Thus, context might include factors relating to the characteristics of the organisational setting, the individual, his or her role in the organisation and the environment (Rousseau 1978). Qualitative studies were excluded but the authors acknowledged that the review would have been enhanced by qualitative literature and also recommended more mixed methods research in this area. The majority of studies had been conducted in the United States, mostly in inpatient settings with some in nursing homes or outpatients.

Kaplan et al. (2010) found that much of the research was methodologically weak and there were conceptual ambiguities, but the overall factors were similar to those found by other authors to describe factors that influence implementation and organisational change, including leadership from top management, organisational culture, data infrastructure and information systems, years involved in quality improvement, physician involvement in quality improvement, microsystems motivation to change, resources for quality improvement and team leadership. Team factors most commonly associated with success in quality improvement were team leadership, group climate, group process, team improvement skills and physician involvement in the team. Of these, team leadership was a particularly strong factor. Whilst this review had recognised limitations, it provided insights into the importance of context in healthcare improvement, which appeared to be just as important as in the manufacturing industry.

The content-context process model

At the same time that Peters and Waterman were exploring the U.S. manufacturing industries, in the United Kingdom, Pettigrew and Whipp (1991) were developing a 'content-context process' model of strategic change from their research exploring why firms operating in the same industry and markets produce different performances across time. They argued that it is necessary to describe both context and process as separate dimensions and stressed the importance of interaction between the components. Rather than a sequenced development, their model suggests that the process of change is a fluid interaction between the nature of the change (the content), conditioning feature (context – both local and national) and the implementation of the change (the actions, reactions and interactions). They suggested that change is built upon a combination of conditioning features (context) and secondary mechanisms (process). Conditioning features include the environment and the state of organisational readiness. Whilst the environment may be clearly tangible; for example, whether there is sufficient technology (diagnostic equipment) to support an improvement, the state of organisational readiness is much less explicit. Pettigrew and Whipp (1991) suggested that there are five factors that determine readiness, including:

- Whether key people are in post
- Whether both the internal and external environments are conducive to the change
- The ability of leadership to create a receptive context that provides the required resources
- The extent to which there is a coherent strategy and
- The change proposal is consistent and integral to the organisation's purpose

Their work describes a generalised state of readiness because, they conclude, the context is dynamic:

> The process by which strategic changes are made seldom moves directly through neat, successive stages of analysis, choice and implementation. Changes in the firm's environment persistently threaten the course and logic of strategic changes.
>
> (Pettigrew and Whipp 1991, p. 31)

Pettigrew and Whipp (1991) therefore concluded that ambiguity is 'one of the defining features of the process, in so far as management action is concerned' (p. 31).

Pettigrew later explored the model within the United Kingdom's National Health Service (NHS) (Pettigrew et al. 1992) where he studied eight matched pairs of NHS organisations (matched as they faced similar agendas but exhibited different outcomes) during the changes that introduced general management during the 1980s. The authors concluded that variations could be explained using a metaphor of receptive and non-receptive contexts for change and they further developed Pettigrew and Whipp's (1991) five factors into eight signs of a receptive context for change (Box 2.1). Despite the promising findings, there have been few attempts to replicate Pettigrew et al.'s model in healthcare. One that did was a study into the use of evidence-based practice in two U.S. hospital nursing departments (Stetler et al. 2007). The research team made qualitative assessments of each department, using the eight signs of receptive context for each case and concluded that the hospital with the highest uptake also had the highest scores of each of Pettigrew et al.'s eight dimensions. Hamilton et al. (2007) also identified a number of aspects of organisational culture that indicated organisational readiness for the introduction of evidence-based multidisciplinary teams within the NHS in the United Kingdom, including stakeholder support and positive past experience of organisational change together with strong team climate.

Whilst Pettigrew et al.'s model has not been explicitly replicated, the underlying findings have been demonstrated repeatedly. Greenhalgh et al. (2004) undertook a systematic review of the healthcare literature on the diffusion of innovations in service organisations on behalf of the UK Department of Health, concluding that there were a number of components with independent but interrelated effects on the change process. They concluded that whilst the

Box 2.1 Signs of receptive context for change

- Quality and coherence of local interpretation of policy
- Availability of key people to lead change (this needs to be across occupational groups and cannot be invested in a single charismatic person)
- A level of external pressure that does not overwhelm the organisation
- A supportive organisational culture
- Effective relations between managers and clinical staff
- Effective networks with local NHS organisations
- Clarity of change goals
- 'Fit' between the change agenda and the local circumstances (noting that some changes will fit and others may not)

Source: Pettigrew, A. et al. *Public Money & Management,* 12, 27–31, 1992.

attention and financial push given to top down programmes were helpful in kick starting innovation, ultimately change was more successful when it was flexible enough to adapt to local circumstances.

First, the nature of the innovation or change (**content**) itself was a factor and in particular, the relative advantage that the potential users perceived it to have was a major determinant of the motivation to make a change. When the innovation was seen to carry risks it was approached more cautiously. However, apparent evidence of the advantage (e.g., evidence-based practice) was not in itself sufficient to create the motivation; the proposed change needed to be compatible with the norms and values of the organisation and the profession together with individual users' values (a receptive **context**).

Greenhalgh et al. (2004) also drew a distinction between different change pathways (**process**) which they described as diffusion (passive spread), dissemination (active and planned efforts to persuade target groups to adopt an innovation), implementation (active and planned efforts to mainstream an innovation) or sustainability (active attempts to make an innovation routine). The distinctions echo Rogers's (1995) categorisation of the way in which the decision to adopt an innovation is made, with the entirely voluntary innovation decision referred to as diffusion and the attempts to influence a group into a consensus innovation decision as dissemination, whilst the more authoritarian innovation decisions are reflected as implementation. In other words, a state of organisational readiness for change can have different degrees of commitment. When organisational readiness for change is high, individuals are more personally motivated and invest more effort in the change process, displaying more persistence in the face of obstacles or setbacks.

In addition to the perception of the relative advantage for the content of the change, Glouberman and Zimmerman (2002) illustrated important distinctions between simple, complicated and complex problems. On reviewing the difference between these, it becomes clear that healthcare problems are invariably complex.

Simple problems: These are predictable with a finite number of variables. Individuals can be given a set of instructions that they follow in a linear manner, and whilst there may be some degree of variation related to experience and expertise, all results fall within predictive and acceptable limits. Cookery recipes are often presented as simple problems.

Complicated problems: These have multiple components but can be broken down into discrete parts that have little interrelation and can be solved by different teams of experts for each part. The parts come together in a predictable manner, and past experience is a good predictor of future performance unless the environment changes. Any untoward event can be broken down and resolved without redesigning the whole. Rocket science is often described as a complicated problem.

Complex problems: In contrast to simple and complicated issues, complex issues are highly variable and the components interact in multiple ways. This means that success in one case does not guarantee success in another. Experience and expertise are a starting point, but the solutions are not linear and need to be carefully calibrated as variable interactions are observed.

In addition to the complexity of healthcare problems, the complexity of the context of healthcare delivery is a compounding factor. As an example, in mental healthcare, Hayward (2012) critically reviewed the applicability of LEAN approaches and identified various challenges in the healthcare context. She argued that engagement in improvement approaches has lagged behind in mental health, in comparison with other healthcare settings. Reasons identified were the complexity of care delivery with multiple agency involvement, the care pathways are less clearly defined and the interaction of acute care providers with different processes and systems. Hayward (2012) highlighted that more integrated care systems would alleviate some of these issues; integrated care and quality improvement are explored in Chapter 3. In a similar study, Whalley et al. (2009) reported that a group of mental health NHS Trusts participating in quality improvement in the south-west of England experienced challenges with medical and organisation-wide engagement. These challenges were potential issues of system-wide culture, leadership and engagement (Hayward 2012).

In England, the NHS Institute for Innovation and Improvement (now discontinued) developed the 'Productive Series' of modules to assist healthcare professionals in service improvement activities using lean principles. In recognition of the varied contexts for improvement activities, the NHS Institute produced different sets of modules for the Productive Ward, the Productive Mental Health Ward, the Productive Community Hospital, the Productive Operating Theatre, Productive Community Services and Productive General Practice. These modules remain available (see http://www.institute.nhs.uk/quality_and_value/ productivity_series/the_productive_series.html).

Mumvuri and Pithouse (2010) reported on their experiences of implementing the NHS Institute for Innovation and Improvement's 'Productive Mental Health Ward' in a mental health trust in London. They discussed preparation for starting the initiative with staff involved from across the organisation and the alignment of the plans with the trust's existing values and objectives. They also visited another NHS trust, but they did not discuss whether there were any contextual differences between the two trusts. They reported on a number of improvements as a result of working through the modules including better organisation of ward resources leading to savings, boards to show patient status (these needed discussion with service use groups with particular concern about confidentiality), increased therapeutic time with nurses (reported in a service user survey) and a reduction on violence and aggression. The authors noted the need to consider how improvements are sustained in the context of organisational changes and other priorities and concluded that factors influencing success of the programme included contextual features such as governance arrangements, senior organisational support and commitment to a bottom-up approach.

In an example that illuminated the importance of engagement at all levels, Greenfield et al. (2011) investigated the factors that shaped the development of interprofessional improvement initiatives in a health organisation in Australia. Six determinants were identified: site receptivity, team issues, leadership, impact on healthcare relations, impact on quality and safety issues, and being institutionally embedded. The organisational commitment was found to be important but was not sufficient if teams were not fully willing to be involved, with issues such as team conflicts, ambivalence, decreasing interest over time and competing work demands being identified by participants and observed by researchers in the field. A local leader ('champion') within the local context supported improvement initiatives, with important features being enthusiasm, positivity, persistence, and the ability to overcome resistance and to engage colleagues. A further theme was relationships, which included collaboration, teamwork, communication, trust, morale and integration of learning opportunities. However, Greenfield et al. (2011) demonstrated that even in environments positively orientated, only half of the improvement initiatives achieved positive progress – indicating that receptivity is only part of the contextual influence.

Culture and climate

The growing recognition that evidence alone cannot predict performance has led to increasing interest in the role of organisational culture. Defining culture remains elusive, but there is a degree of consensus that it is a condition generated by a collective set of assumptions held by a group of people and which directs their perceptions and behaviours. Culture will therefore influence the extent to which individuals perceive that a change (improvement) is desirable and possible and is a key element of determining the receptivity of a context.

Assessing culture is complex, and Schein (1996) described how culture manifests itself at three levels:

1   The tacit assumptions, which people may or may not be aware of
2   The espoused values: what the group feels *should* be driving the organisation and how it wants to present itself publicly
3   The actual daily practices that result from the complex integration of the espoused values, the deeper assumptions and the immediate requirements of the situation

The potential for contradiction among the three levels can lead to inconsistencies and means that caution should be applied before using espoused values as a diagnostic for assessing the receptivity of a given context.

Organisational culture and climate reflect different aspects of this trilogy. Organisational climate is defined as the group members' conscious perceptions of the practices and procedures, whereas culture is defined as the shared assumptions and values (Schneider et al. 2013). As such climate can be measured with relative ease, for example by using the cultural barometer (Rafferty et al. 2015). Climate measures can be helpful as conscious perceptions can drive the socialisation of new members. However, if the members' perceptions are not aligned with the tacit assumptions of the culture in practice, any measures may fail to adequately reflect the receptivity of a given improvement project.

Schein (1996) also described how perception of the culture can differ among individuals at different places within the organisation. The operators who perform the work of the organisation may have different assumptions from the engineers who design the work processes, and they may differ from the executives who set the strategy. In healthcare, the multiplicity of professions can mean their different subcultures are also very disparate. Following the public inquiry into healthcare failings at Mid-Staffordshire NHS Foundation Trust in England, Francis (2013) found that different professions having discipline-specific codes could lead to a 'separation of cultural identity between different groups' and that NHS staff must remember that they are part of one large team with one objective: 'the proper care and treatment of their patients' (p. 1401). The espoused values for the NHS are embedded in the NHS Constitution, which was first published by the Department of Health (DH) in 2009 (current version, DH 2015). Reflecting Schein's distinction between espoused culture and culture in practice, Francis observed that the NHS Constitution intends to set out:

> a common source of values and principles by which the NHS works, but it has not as yet had the impact it should. It should become the common reference point for all staff. [...] All staff should be required to commit to abiding by its values and principles.
>
> (Francis 2013, Vol. 3, p. 1399)

Commonly, healthcare organisations publish their own set of values aimed at their workforce but again, the actual daily practice across the organisation and within different groups of staff may differ from these espoused values.

Receptive contexts are those in which there is a high degree of alignment on perceptions, both between people in different professions and at different positions in the hierarchy, and also high alignment among tacit assumptions, espoused behaviours and daily practice. Alignment may be more important in successful quality improvement than content and modifying a large-scale project to align with local cultures may be more effective than trying to replicate success in other places faithfully in different contexts.

Organisational readiness for change

Quality improvement is a form of organisational change, and Weiner (2009) considers that organisational readiness is a necessary precondition to change, with increasing importance as change becomes more complex. Weiner's (2009) 'Organisational readiness to change' theory sets out that readiness is a collective state shared by the organisation's members, whilst varied perceptions among staff members indicates a lack of shared readiness. Readiness is also specific to a given change effect and thus an organisation may have high readiness for one change but not for another (Weiner 2009).

Weiner (2009) suggested that structural readiness and psychological readiness are interrelated and that staff take into consideration the organisation's structural assets and deficits in deciding whether they believe that change is both desirable and achievable; not only do they decide whether the change is desirable, but also whether they believe whether it is possible. The presence of generalised organisational resources (physical and cultural) that might be termed as a generic receptive context creates a capacity or, as Weiner terms it, change valence, which influences but does not wholly determine organisational readiness. This capacity needs to be considered together with situational factors specific to a given change initiative and because of this, organisational readiness for change is situational rather than a general state of affairs:

> The content of change matters as much as the context of change. A healthcare organization could, for example, exhibit a culture that values risk-taking and experimentation, a positive working environment (e.g., good managerial-clinical relationships), and a history of successful change implementation. Yet, despite this receptive context, this organization could still exhibit a high readiness to implement electronic medical records, but a low readiness to implement an open-access scheduling system. Commitment is, in part, change specific.
>
> (Weiner 2009, p. 70)

As Weiner illustrates, individuals may believe that two changes are desirable but that only one is feasible within the organisation. Thus, as well as assessing the structural readiness, the psychological readiness of the individuals who will need to enact the change must be understood. On the one hand, individuals could be confident that the organisational context would allow a change to be successful but show little or no motivation to do so, and on the other hand, they might be strongly motivated but lack confidence that it can be achieved. Individuals might also be at any point of the continuum in-between. Organisational readiness will be highest when organisational members both want to implement an organisational change and also feel confident that the organisational structures will allow it. The role of the quality improvement leader is therefore both to assess the current state of readiness and to take action in order to motivate individuals and give them confidence that the organisation's structures will facilitate the change.

Box 2.2 summarises a study that used Weiner's (2009) theory to develop a better understanding of the barriers and facilitators to implementing the World Health Organisation (WHO) 'Ten Steps to successful breastfeeding' across several U.S. hospitals (Nickel et al. 2013).

There is also a temporal aspect to organisational readiness. Reay et al. (2006) found that there are windows of opportunity contingent on the organisation's needs and the external

---

Box 2.2 Understanding the barriers and facilitators to improvement: Application of Weiner's (2009) 'Organisational Readiness to Change' theory

This qualitative study investigated the barriers and facilitators to implementing the World Health Organisation (WHO) 'Ten Steps to Successful Breastfeeding' across eight U.S. hospitals, a complex change that required collaboration across staff from multiple disciplines in various units. The interviews, conducted with a range of staff across the different organisations, revealed many important contextual factors. For example, attitudes, beliefs and practices varied across day and night shifts, and management support was perceived as influencing the collective commitment to implement the Ten Steps. A further factor was staffing levels, which were considered sometimes inadequate to provide the support needed, and visitors in the room were perceived as having a negative effect on women trying to breastfeed. A mapping of the factors identified across the eight hospitals highlighted some variations. For example, the issue of visitors in the room was considered an influence at just three of the eight hospitals; staffing levels were a factor at five hospitals, but differences between night and day shifts were raised at seven hospitals. The authors highlighted that the size of the hospital seemed to affect a number of factors identified.

The authors argued that, based on their results, other hospitals would benefit from conducting a context-specific baseline assessment of organisational level factors impacting on collective efficacy and/or collective commitment to achieving the Ten Steps. They highlighted that the factors may vary across contexts. They suggested that having identified the factors, multilevel, context-specific strategies can be developed to increase commitment and efficacy. They also highlighted that strategies successful in one context may not be in another.

Source: Nickel, N.C. et al., *Midwifery*, 29, 956–964, 2013.

climate. In their study looking at introducing new work roles, they observed that successful managers were able to consider the timeliness of change and 'fit' the new role by presenting and classifying the role in such a way as to make it congruent with existing practice and organisational structures. Similarly, Shekelle et al. (2010) evaluated five safety interventions for the U.S. Agency for Healthcare Research and Quality (AHRQ) and concluded that safety improvement is not a single-shot intervention but a series of actions that evolve over time as a result of their interactions with the context over time. This suggests that a single theory of how context impacts quality improvement would be too simplistic.

Assessing organisational readiness

By definition then, organisational readiness assessment for change (quality improvement or innovation) is dependent on local factors and cannot be reduced to a single list of attributes or checklist. There are, however, a number of tools that help to direct the assessment, including:

- The Promoting Action on Research Implementation in Health Services (PARiHS) model (Kitson et al. 2008)
- The Context Assessment Index (CAI) (McCormack et al. 2009)
- The Organisational Readiness to Change Assessment (ORCA) (Helfrich et al. 2009)

The PARiHS framework is a specific healthcare adaptation of Pettigrew and Whipp's model and is based on three core elements that predict the extent to which implementation of new evidence will be implemented: (1) the strength and nature of the evidence as perceived by multiple stakeholders, (2) the quality of the context or environment in which the research is implemented and (3) the processes by which implementation is facilitated. Both the CAI and the ORCA are attempts to apply Kitson et al.'s (2008) PARiHS model in local contexts.

The CAI, a 37-item instrument, measures general readiness for research utilisation, rather than readiness for implementation of a specific, discrete practice change. The ORCA has 19 subscales and seeks to focus on particular projects. Both the CAI and ORCA require further validation before the results could be generalised and used to compare organisations, but both serve as useful aide-memoires for quality improvement leaders at a practice level.

Instead of quantifying context as an objective and independent reality, Weick (1995) preferred to look at sense-making within organisations. Sense-making is the way in which people frame their experience to make it meaningful. Organisational sense-making is the way in which a particular frame or lens to view things becomes dominant and becomes a shared awareness and understanding. Weick's work has provided insight, particularly into the ways in which organisations make sense of unexpected or ambiguous situations and emphasises the dynamic, impermanent nature of contexts. As Weick argues:

> The basic idea of sense making is that reality is an ongoing accomplishment that emerges from efforts to create order and make retrospective sense of what occurs.

> (Weick 1993, p. 635)

This is particularly important in contexts where there is a high level of ambiguity and fluidity and where the past is not a reliable indicator of the present or future. For example, the demands on emergency departments are unpredictable and one serious accident can quickly change the whole context of the working environment. In this situation, context needs to be understood in real time with rapid sense-making based on imperfect data to create a sense of order that allows for decision-making. Weick and Sutcliffe (2007) went on to develop their theory of High Reliability Organisations, highlighting the need for collective mindfulness of the context in real time rather than on shared understanding of history. Chapter 7 considers High Reliability Organisations in detail.

Ethnography as a way of understanding context

The unspoken assumptions that shape culture and therefore shape organisational readiness cannot be directly measured, and discerning them requires qualitative investigation methods. Ethnography is a well-established qualitative research methodology and there is increasing interest in its application in healthcare as a way of understanding context and culture for care. More recently, there has been recognition of how ethnography might enable healthcare professionals to better understand the context for improvement.

Hammersley (2007) asserted that there is no standardised definition of ethnography due to the way that it evolved with multiple disciplinary influences. He traced the origins of ethnography to nineteenth century anthropology, where it usually involved the detailed description of a culture or a community, and then during the twentieth century, it started being used as a research method within sociology. Hammersley (2007) set out what ethnography involves: the participation in people's everyday lives over an extended period of time, observing, listening, asking questions and collecting documents and artefacts, 'gathering whatever data are available to threw light on the issues that are the line of inquiry' (p. 3). Key features are that there are usually multiple data sources, inquiry is unstructured and exploratory, and the focus is on in-depth study of a few cases or just one in the natural setting.

Savage (2000) identified that ethnography is considered contextual and reflexive, helping to uncover meanings of people's actions and words, rather than measuring them. She argued for the greater use of ethnography as a research methodology in healthcare for the study of everyday settings and investigation of beliefs and practices within the context that they occur. There is a well-established use of ethnography within healthcare, particularly nursing, though its use is usually adapted from the traditional ways developed by sociologists, which required lengthy immersion in the field and may not be feasible where the goal is to inform practice development and rapid improvement. However, Savage (2000) highlighted the use of 'focused ethnography', where researchers enter the field with more focused research questions and emphasise participant observation less. Observation (which may occur on a continuum of complete participant to complete observer, depending on the role undertaken) does, however, remain a core feature of ethnography and may be unstructured or more purposeful. As an example, Taylor et al. (2015) conducted a focused ethnographic study of the care of older people in an emergency department, which used non-participant observation and semi-structured interviews.

Dixon-Woods (2003) highlighted that ethnographers face various difficulties in practice, for example, observing is not always comfortable, and there can be ethical issues encountered, particularly if care observed is suboptimal. However, she argued that that such issues can and should be overcome as ethnography's potential to contribute to safety and quality in healthcare has been underexploited. She considered that ethnography is especially helpful for areas where issues are sensitive and multifaceted, and can help to uncover the tacit rather than obvious:

> It can capture the winks, sighs, head shaking, and gossip that may be exceptionally powerful in explaining why mistakes happen, but which more formal methods will miss.

(Dixon-Woods 2003, pp. 326–327)

She goes on to describe how Taxis and Barber's (2003) ethnographic study of intravenous medication errors in healthcare led to insights that would not have otherwise been uncovered.

Ethnography has been identified as potentially enabling better understanding of the professional, organisational and cultural aspects of context and has been used for gaining understanding of context in a range of healthcare quality improvement areas (Leslie et al. 2014). However, although Leslie et al. (2014) described ethnography as being established as a 'powerful method for understanding healthcare contexts' (p. 100), they also warned about the challenges of 'importing' a qualitative research methodology from the social sciences into the quality improvement field. They asserted that ethnographers must be transparent about how they collect and interpret their data. The need for researchers to be reflexive about their role and influence on data is well recognised as promoting trustworthiness of qualitative findings (Baillie 2015). As an example of good practice, a report of an ethnographic study of factors affecting medication adherence included a section on reflexivity, explaining that the researcher kept a journal to express thoughts, feelings and frustrations separately from the observation field notes, reducing their influence on the data (Ens et al. 2014).

There are many examples where use of ethnographic methods within healthcare research has led to more in-depth understandings about context and factors that influence the quality of care. For example, person-centred care is considered to be ideal for people with dementia (Edwardsson et al. 2010), but there are difficulties in applying these principles in hospital settings and improving care (Dewing and Dijk 2014). Clissett et al. (2013) reported on a qualitative study that used observation and interviews to explore the potential for hospital care of people with dementia to be more person-centred. The study was set in two different hospitals and a variety of wards. The data were analysed using Kitwood's (1997) model of personhood (identity, attachment, comfort, inclusion and occupation) to uncover examples of good practice and also areas where there was potential for improvement. The researchers concluded that person-centred care needed to be valued by the organisation, teams and individuals, for care of people with dementia to improve in acute hospital settings. In a further example, Taylor et al.'s (2015) study illuminated that the time-pressured, high-speed emergency department environment and a culture that focused on priority setting and throughput of patients did not fit well with older people and their complex needs, and put them at risk of sub-standard care. The study findings highlighted how emergency department culture was a barrier to nurses who desired to provide high-quality care for older people.

In another example, Ens et al. (2014) identified that the focus on studies into medication adherence has often been on the patients alone, but their study included factors surrounding the patient through observation of patients, physicians and pharmacists in pharmacies and physicians' offices, as well as conducting interviews. They argued that adherence to medication needs to be investigated from the cultural perspectives of the patient as well as the healthcare providers and healthcare systems so that improvement interventions integrate the various perspectives with the healthcare system. The observations offered insight into the context for the flow of patients through the physicians' office and pharmacies and also how non-English speaking patients were managed. The study highlighted the importance of including family members in the care of South Asian people as patients rarely attended appointments alone and their family members also learned about the cardiac medications and were involved in helping them to take them. The family members were used as facilitators/translators for the patient and helped to culturally contextualise information provided by the professionals. The quality of the provider–patient relationship was a further important influence on adherence to healthcare; physicians being patient and non-judgmental about lapses in adherence positively affected relationship building. The observations also revealed that language barriers were less of a challenge in the visits to physicians than the pharmacies, as family members more often accompanied non-English-speaking patients to physician visits than to pharmacists and physicians also often spoke the patient's language.

Whilst recognising the potential benefits of ethnography for quality improvement, Leslie et al. (2014) identified key differences between traditional ethnography and quality and safety research in terms of mission, form and scale:

- **Mission**: Traditional ethnographers aim to describe and critically analyse power and social relations within the environment whilst in quality and safety research, the goal is to describe and feedback the perspectives gained for improvement purposes.

- **Form:** Ethnographers traditionally undertook long-term exposure to the environment as a way of increasing the quality of the data collected, but in quality improvement research, rapid results are usually required.

- **Scale:** In ethnography, researchers traditionally developed in-depth accounts of the social context on one site, but in quality improvement, a multisite approach may be intended. However, in a study that Leslie et al. (2014) described as 'pioneering', ethnographic methods were used across multiple sites ($n = 19$), leading to insights into contextual issues affecting improvement activities (see Box 2.3).

Leslie et al. (2014) went on to explain how their team's ethnographic field researchers have developed long-term relationships with four ICUs and their staff where they are collecting high-quality data. As with any adapted use of a research methodology, what is important is clarity about how adaptations have occurred and the rationale for these.

Box 2.3 Case study – What counts?

Dixon-Woods et al. (2012) used ethnographic methods to study the introduction of a national programme (Matching Michigan) in the UK NHS to reduce central venous line associated bacteraemia infections in intensive care units (ICUs). A key element of this programme was the central reporting of infections, which was anticipated to create peer pressure to improve practice and eliminate infections.

There was mixed motivation within the ICUs, with some seeing the reporting as performance monitoring rather than quality improvement; however, the researchers found no evidence that there was 'gaming' or deliberate attempts to skew the data. What they did discover was that, despite a nationally defined data set, what counted was highly context specific.

They found three separate methods of data collection. In the first method, the ICUs collected the required information as part of each individual patient's clinical record, although this differed with nurses completing the form in certain units and junior doctors in others. At the end of each month, the study controller for each unit reviewed the forms of any patient with a possible infection, calling up the microbiology results

(Continued)

Box 2.3 Case study – What counts? (*Continued*)

as required. In the second method, infection control nurses who were not part of the ICU team visited the ICU daily and reviewed records and discussed cases with the unit staff and then recorded possible infections. At the end of the month, the study controller received microbiology data and the infection control nurses' reports. In the third method, designated ICU staff (nurses or doctors) conducted a daily census which was reviewed at the end of the month by the study controller. Some units counted the central line infections by patient (any patient unlucky enough to have more than one infection site was still counted as one site), whereas other units counted each infection, even if in the same patient. All units used a degree of professional judgement to determine whether a positive blood culture was attributable to the central line.

The choice of method was determined in part by the resources available. Larger units could assign data collectors who had received training to ensure consistency but smaller units were more likely to rely on whoever was looking after the patient that day. There were also differences in the laboratory processes and the extent to which microbiologists were able to be involved in clinical decision-making. Some units had microbiologists who attended clinical rounds, whilst others gave advice only when asked. The difference in data collection and input to clinical decision-making meant that the study controllers in each ICU had different data on which to decide whether a central line–associated bacteraemia had occurred and therefore the data reported nationally was not consistent.

Conclusion

This chapter has explored the nature of context and how it refers to both physical environment and structures and to the perception, attitudes and assumptions that influence how people will react to the improvement intervention. Context is more than a static backdrop to quality improvement; it comprises a highly complex set of features that interact with the evidence-based content of an improvement intervention, changing the way it is implemented and influencing the success of the improvement. Those seeking to make improvements in quality need to be aware of the impact of local contexts on their project and be mindful that successes in other places are unlikely to be replicated without attention to the need for local modification.

Improvement leaders should seek methods to assess the context and to align all aspects of context such that there is an organisational readiness for the specific improvement. Standardised tools to assist the assessment of organisational readiness may play a useful role but more qualitative methods of exploring less overt aspects of context can uncover important factors within the context that could be critical to the ultimate success of an improvement initiative. Whilst local improvement projects are unlikely to undertake detailed ethnographic methods, the findings from research evaluations, together with surveys and checklists can frame the improvement leader's thinking and help them to develop working hypotheses which can be quickly checked out in order to ensure organisational readiness for the improvement intervention.

References

Baillie, L. (2015) Scientific rigour in qualitative research. *Nursing Standard* 29(46): 36–42.

Clissett, P., Porock, D., Harwood, R.H., and Gladman, J.R.F. (2013) The challenges of achieving person-centred care in acute hospitals. *International Journal of Nursing Studies* 50: 1495–1503.

Department of Health (2015) *The NHS Constitution for England*. Available from: https://www.gov.uk/government/publications/the-nhs-constitution-for-england (accessed on 9 January 2017).

Dewing, J., and Dijk, S. (2014) What is the current state of care for older people with dementia in general hospitals? A literature review. *Dementia* (published online 23 January 2014).

Dixon-Woods, M. (2003) What can ethnography do for quality and safety in healthcare? *Quality and Safety in Health Care* 12: 326–327.

Dixon Woods, M., Bion, J., and Tarrant, C. (2012) What counts? An ethnographic study of infection data reported to a patient safety program. *Milbank Quarterly* 90(3): 548–591.

Edwardsson, D., Fetherstonhaugh, D., and Nay, R. (2010) Promoting a continuation of self and normality: Person-centred care as described by people with dementia, their family members and aged care staff. *Journal of Clinical Nursing* 19: 2611–2618.

Ens, T.A., Seneviratne, C.C., Jones, C., and King-Shier, K.M. (2014) Factors influencing medication adherence in South Asian people with cardiac disorders: An ethnographic study. *International Journal of Nursing Studies* 51: 1472–1481.

Francis, R. (2013) *Report of the Mid Staffordshire NHS Foundation Trust – Public Inquiry*. Available from: http://www.midstaffspublicinquiry.com/report

Glouberman, S. and Zimmerman, B. (2002) Complicated and complex systems: What would successful reform of Medicare look like? *Romanow Papers* 2: 21–53.

Greenfield, D., Nugus, P., Travaglia, J., and Braithwaite, J. (2011) Factors that shape the development of interprofessional improvement initiatives in health organisation. *BMJ Quality and Safety* 20: 332–337.

Greenhalgh, T., Robert, G., MacFarlane, F., Bate, P., and Kyriakidou, O. (2004) Diffusion of innovations in service organizations: Systematic review and recommendations. *Milbank Quarterly* 82(4): 581–629.

Hamilton, S., McLaren, S., and Mulhall, A. (2007) Assessing organisational readiness for change: Use of diagnostic analysis prior to the implementation of a multidisciplinary assessment for acute stroke care. *Implementation Science* 2: 21. Available from: http://www.implementationscience.com/content/2/1/21

Hammersley, M. (2007) *Ethnography: Principles in Practice*, 3rd edn. Abingdon: Routledge.

Hayward, L.M. (2012) How applicable is lean in mental health? A critical appraisal. *International Journal of Clinical Leadership* 17: 165–173.

Helfrich, C., Li, Y., Sharp, N., and Sales, A. (2009) Organizational readiness to change assessment (ORCA): Development of an instrument based on the Promoting Action on Research in Health Services (PARIHS) framework. *Implement Science* 4(38): 38.

Kaplan, H.C., Brady, P.W., Dritz, M.C., Hooper, D.K., Linam, W.M., Froehle, C.M., and Margolis, P. (2010) The influence of context in quality improvement success in healthcare: A systematic review of the literature. *Millbank Quarterly* 88(4): 500–559.

Kirchner, J.E., Parker, L.E., Bonner, L.M., Fickel, J.J., Yano, E.M., and Ritchie, M.J. (2012) Roles of managers, frontline staff and local champions. In Implementing quality improvement: Stakeholders' perspectives. *Journal of Evaluation in Clinical Practice* 18: 63–69.

Kitson, A. L., Ryecroft-Malone, J., Harvey, G., McCormack, B., Seers, K., and Titchen, A. (2008) Evaluating the successful implementation of evidence into practice using the PARIHS framework: Theoretical and practical challenges. *Implementation Science* 3:1. Available from: http://www.implementationscience.com/content/3/1/1

Kitwood, T. (1997) *Dementia Reconsidered: The Person Comes First*. Buckingham: Open University Press.

Leslie, M., Paradis, E., Gropper, M.A., Reeves, S., and Kitto, S. (2014) Applying ethnography to the study of context in healthcare quality and safety. *BMJ Quality and Safety* 23: 99–105.

McCormack B., McCarthy G., Wright J., and Coffey A. (2009) Development and testing of the Context Assessment Index (CAI). *Worldviews on Evidence-Based Nursing* 6(1):27–35.

Mumvuri, M. and Pithouse, A. (2010) Implementing and evaluating the productive ward initiative in a mental health trust. *Nursing Times* 106(41): 15–18.

Nickel, N.C., Taylor, E.C., Labbok, M.H., Weiner, B.J., and Williamson, N.E. (2013) Applying organisational theory to understand barriers and facilitators to the implementation of baby-friendly: A multisite qualitative study. *Midwifery* 29: 956–964.

Øvretveit, J., Bate, P., Cleary, P., Cretin, S., Gustafson, D., McInnes, K., et al. (2002) Quality collaboratives: Lessons from research. *Quality and Safety in Health Care* 11(4): 345–351.

Peters, T., and Waterman, R. (1982) *In Search of Excellence: Lessons from America's Best-Run Corporations*. New York, NY: Warner.

Pettigrew, A., Ferlie, E., and McKee, L. (1992) Shaping strategic change-the case of the NHS in the 1980s. *Public Money and Management* 12(3): 27–31.

Pettigrew, A.M. and Whipp, R. (1991) *Managing Change for Competitive Success*. Oxford: Blackwell.

Rafferty, A.M., Philippou, J., Fitzpatrick, J.M., and Ball, J. (2015) *Culture of Care Barometer*. London: National Nursing Research Unit. Available from: https://www.england.nhs.uk/wp-content/uploads/2015/03/culture-care-barometer.pdf. (accessed on 9 January 2017)

Reay, T., Golden-Biddle, K., and Germann, K. (2006) Legitimizing a new role: Small wins and micro processes of change. *Academy of Management Journal* 49(5): 977–998.

Rogers, E.M. (1995) *Diffusion of Innovations*. New York, NY: Free Press.

Rousseau, D.M. (1978) Characteristics of departments, positions and individuals: Context for attitudes and behaviour. *Administrative Science Quarterly* 23: 521–540.

Savage, J. (2000) Ethnography and healthcare. *British Medical Journal* 321: 1400–1402.

Schein, E. (1996) Three cultures of management: The key to organizational learning. *MIT Sloan Management Review* 38(1): 9.

Schneider, B., Ehrhart, M.G., and Macey, W.H. (2013) Organizational climate and culture. *Annual Review of Psychology* 64: 361–388.

Self, D., and Schraeder, M. (2009) Enhancing the success of organizational change: Matching readiness strategies with sources of resistance. *Leadership and Organization Development Journal* 30(2): 167–182.

Shekelle, P., Pronovost, P., Wachter, R., Taylor, L., Dy, S., Foy, R., Hempel, S., McDonald, K., Øvretveit, J., and Rubenstein, L. (2010) *Assessing the Evidence for Context-Sensitive Effectiveness and Safety of Patient Safety Practices: Developing Criteria*. Prepared under Contract No. HHSA-290-2009-10001C, pp. 1–76.

Stetler, C.B., Ritchie, J., Rycroft-Malone, J., Schultz, A., and Charns, M. (2007) Improving quality of care through routine, successful implementation of evidence-based practice at the bedside: An organizational case study protocol using the Pettigrew and Whipp model of strategic change. *Implementation Science* 2: 3. Available from: http://www.implementationscience.com/contents/2/1/3

Taxis, K., and Barber, N. (2003) Causes of intravenous medication errors: An ethnographic study. *Quality and Safety in Healthcare* 12: 236–237.

Taylor, R.J., Rush, K.L., and Robinson, C.A. (2015) Nurses' experiences of caring for the older adult in the emergency department: A focused ethnography. *International Emergency Nursing* 23: 185–189.

Weick, K. (1993) The collapse of sensemaking in organizations: The Mann Gulch disaster. *Administrative Science Quarterly* 3: 628–652.

Weick, K. (1995) *Sensemaking in Organizations (Foundations for Organizational Science)*. Thousand Oaks, CA: Sage.

Weick K. and Sutcliffe K. (2007) *Managing the Unexpected: Resilient Performance in an Age of Uncertainty*. San Francisco, CA: Jossey Bass.

Weiner, B.J. (2009) A theory of organisational readiness for change. *Implementation Science* 4: 67

Whalley, P., Rayment, J., and Cooke, M. (2009) The redesign practices and capabilities of NHS Trusts in England: A snapshot study. *International Journal of Healthcare Technology and Management* 10(4–5): 340–359.

3 System Improvement

Elaine Maxwell, Lesley Baillie and Jerusha Murdoch-Kelly

Introduction

Healthcare is increasingly complex and delivered through different though linked services and in different places in order to address the multiple health needs of the population. Providers of healthcare are becoming more diverse, with main providers outsourcing parts of the service to third parties. In particular, many people are living with more than one and often several long-term health conditions. Their care management will include access to a range of community services as well as hospital-based care, delivered by multi-professional teams, who work collaboratively with patients, families and communities. In this environment, care delivery (as well as the care itself) is becoming more complex and in order to make improvements, we need to understand the system in which care is provided.

This chapter will explain systems theory with application to healthcare practice and improvement. The chapter will include discussion of LEAN principles within the context of systems thinking and also considers how systems are nested within larger systems and the need to establish the boundaries of the systems when undertaking improvement. The chapter also highlights how teams, as microsystems, play an essential role within improvement activity, as the larger system cannot otherwise improve. For many patients, especially those with multiple comorbidities, involving care requires integration of microsystems and so different types and levels of integration will be reviewed. Finally, the chapter will examine interprofessional collaborative working and provide examples related to quality improvement in healthcare.

Objectives

This chapter's objectives are to:

- Explore systems theory with application to practice
- Examine LEAN thinking with application to healthcare systems
- Discuss improvement in the context of microsystems
- Consider improvement within integrated care and across organisational boundaries
- Discuss collaborative interprofessional working in relation to quality improvement

Introduction to systems theory

Much improvement work takes place around specific problems which are considered in isolation. Vincent and Amalberti (2016) noted that the most dramatic quality improvements reported in healthcare have been those focused on a single core clinical issue and a narrow timescale or improving the reliability of a single pathway. In many cases, the evidence base is clear and overwhelming and remains constant in any situation. For example, hand hygiene is a universal principle of quality improvement and applies in all healthcare situations regardless of the system. However, whilst some very focused projects can undoubtedly be highly successful, much of healthcare is complex (not just complicated) and can only be improved through an understanding of the system in which care is provided. Schein (2013) noted that:

> the world is becoming more technologically complex, interdependent, and culturally diverse, which makes the building of relationships more and more necessary to get things accomplished and, at the same time, more difficult. (p. 62)

This is evident as life expectancy rises and the number of people with two or more long-term conditions increases. As the patients' needs become more complex, challenges to the traditional disease- or organ-based pathway approach to quality improvement arise as what works for one disease may not produce the same outcomes for a person with comorbidities. Long-term conditions also mean that healthcare is provided to the same patient at multiple locations and different times. Without consideration of these other factors, interventions for a single element have a much lower probability of success. Not only is there a risk that the intervention will be less successful, but there is the possibility of an unintended consequence elsewhere in the system. Complexity is not necessarily unmanageable, rather understanding how it emerges and how it impacts the pre-existing relationships within the system determines whether increasing complexity damages or enhances the system. Thus, care for people with long-term conditions must be studied as a whole rather than reduced to a series of discrete sections.

Deming and Edwards (1993) described the four lenses which collectively lead to profound knowledge about improvement. The first lens is appreciation of a system, and understanding how relationships between different parts of a system can facilitate or unintentionally restrict the way in which the individual elements work. Deming and Edwards concluded that, for organisations, it is ultimately the working of the system, rather than the actions of individuals, that determines the quality of output. Quality improvement therefore must be considered within the relevant system theory and in some cases, improvement can only happen when the system is redesigned.

Background to systems theory

Seddon and Caulkin (2007) described a system, at its simplest, as being an entity that adds up to more than the sum of its constituent parts. Systems come in different forms; they can be naturally occurring, an engineered system or sociological. Systems thinking is about 'joined-up-ness', and it can be argued that quality failures are due to managing the parts rather than the whole.

Interest in systems emerged in natural sciences and mathematics as a reaction to the post Enlightenment paradigm in which the dominant method of study was to reduce phenomena into separate elements and then study each component individually. Problems or areas of interest are characterised as isolated parts of a process and are resolved without reference to any other processes or the context that they sit within. In contrast, systems theory explores a phenomenon as part of a set of interrelated or interdependent elements within a particular environment that interact with each other (intentionally or otherwise) leading to system-wide outcomes. It draws on a number of different academic disciplines, starting with von Bertalanffy's (1968) Theory of Systems in which he described the system as a sort of 'gestalt' where the whole equals more than the sum of the parts:

> the scientific exploration of wholes and wholeness which, not so long ago were considered metaphysical notions transcending the countries of science.
>
> (von Bertalanffy 1968, p. xviii)

Bertalanffy described systems in physical terms, using metaphors from mathematics and biology. He proposed structured methods of inquiry that assume that there is an independent, objective reality of systems in the world that could be empirically measured. Designing systems is based on identifying physical resources required, identifying the actions to be taken and then following a protocol. Checkland (1999), however, made a distinction between the elements of systems that are characterised by physical structures and visible processes (which he described as hard systems) and the important but less tangible aspects of systems that are not as well defined and those that people may not even be consciously aware of but none the less have a significant impact and are usually socio-economic (which he describes as soft systems). Soft systems approaches assume that organisational problems are 'messy' and that there is no objective reality so stakeholders interpret problems differently and that understanding humans' behaviour is critical to understanding how a system performs. Exploring and improving soft systems involves understanding how decisions are made and how the relationships between different parts of the system impact that decision-making. The complexity of soft systems means that assessing and improving them requires a high level of discretion and cannot be codified into a generalised protocol. Forrester (1971) developed system dynamics as a mathematical modelling technique to help understand the nonlinear, dynamic behaviour of complex systems. The model recognises that any system has feedback loops (often circular) that modify behaviour and computers are used to model large amounts of data to describe the relationships. Soft systems approaches have been developed by social science and management disciplines and have led to a move to interpretative methods of inquiry.

Senge (1990) called systems thinking 'the fifth discipline' that integrates the four pillars of personal mastery, models, shared vision and team learning. He asserted that system thinking is what creates a learning organisation, one that is flexible and responsive:

> Systems thinking is a discipline for seeing 'structures' that underlie complex situations and for discerning high from low leverage change. That is, by seeing whole we learn to foster health. To do so, systems thinking offers a language that begins to begin restructuring how we think.
>
> (Senge 1990, p. 69)

Systems as a whole comprise both hard and soft systems and healthcare improvement requires the integration of both. The World Health Organisation (WHO) Surgical Checklist is an exemplar of this (see Box 3.1). The hard system approach to the prevalence of 'never events' in surgery was reviewed and led to the design of a system with physical resources (checklists) and actions (huddles). Initial trials saw significant reduction in adverse events in operating theatres but early successes have not been easily replicated. There are plenty of examples of where teams have 'gone through the motion' of the checklist without any regard to the soft systems simultaneously in play.

Box 3.1 WHO Surgical Checklist

In 2007, the World Health Organisation (WHO) started a programme to identify minimum standards to eliminate errors associated with surgery. The resulting checklist vertically integrates a system which reflects the patient's journey. The three sections (sign in, time-out and sign out) each consider the immediate actions but also check that the whole system is functioning. The sign in happens preanaesthetic and the staff check not only the anaesthetic issues but that the patient has consented and that the operation and site are clearly understood. In the time-out before the first incision, the operating theatre team check not only that they are prepared, but that other parts of the system have also prepared, for example whether blood has been made available for transfusion. When the surgery is completed, the sign out includes not only review of the process (including swab counts) but checking that the next phase, the post-operative care, is understood and adequately resourced. The checklist also incorporates horizontal system integration, requiring anaesthetists, surgeons, nurses and operating theatre practitioners to reflect on the system together.

The checklist was piloted in eight hospitals across different parts of the world with very different contexts. Haynes et al. (2011) demonstrated that introduction of the checklist was associated with a reduction in complication rates from 11% during the baseline period to 7% following implementation. The authors comment:

> The improvement in outcomes did not correlate consistently with improvements in specific processes of care, suggesting that an intervening mechanism was at work. (p. 105)

This suggests that using a systems approach to improvement has an effect that is over and above the improvement in the individual components. Scepticism about the WHO checklist has grown as the original improvements have failed to be replicated. However, Van Klei et al. (2012) found that the reductions in errors and mortality were strongly related to completion of all sections of the checklist. In the United Kingdom, Pickering et al. (2013) observed 294 operations in 5 hospitals and reported that whilst time-out was attempted 87% of the time, this dropped to 8.8% for sign out. Implementation of the surgical safety checklist clearly requires a full understanding of the system by the whole team.

Systems thinking in practice

Systems theory has been used in a wide range of industries to understand how safety failures occur. Learning from aviation, rail services and nuclear power has repeatedly shown the benefits of system-based approaches to improvement. Reason (1997) used systems theory to develop his 'Swiss cheese' model (see also Chapter 1). Reason suggested that the system has numerous hazards that may be managed at a component level by barriers and when viewed at that level they may appear to be effective and appropriate controls. These component barriers can be inherently weakened by other aspects of the system and create a hole in the defence. As with the holes in Swiss cheese, these weaknesses may not be apparent from outside but when they are aligned, the hazard can pass through and result in an adverse event. Vincent et al. (2000) developed this model for healthcare, producing the London protocol for examining the systems factors that contribute to patient safety incidents.

Much of the empirical work on systems improvement in healthcare to date has focused on retrospective analysis of adverse events and a growing interest in the contribution of human factors and ergonomics. There has been some suggestion that rules can be imposed to reduce human variability and that this would keep the system safe, but Dekker (2007) called for a move beyond attempts to manage the future based on past errors and recognising that open systems are fluid and ever changing. Open systems, such as healthcare have uncontrolled influences and are constantly evolving meaning that new, unanticipated properties can emerge. Whilst examination of historical error can reveal the relationships between diverse elements of systems, and patterns can be identified, open systems can only be partially managed and improved, meaning that certainty can never be assured. It is therefore important to be alert to emergent relationships within the system.

Hollnagel et al. (2013) described systems safety management as falling into two categories: Safety-I and Safety-II:

Safety-1 is the absence of actual accidents or incidents and it assumes that the system can be studied in constituent parts. It also assumes that safety is a binary construct: it is either present or absent with no grey areas. This does not recognise the latent risks that Reason's Swiss cheese model addresses and the absence of incidents may be due to luck rather than design. Slight changes to the system may weaken the defence barriers and a catastrophic accident may occur. Safety-1 may be somewhat like playing Russian roulette: the hazard may not be realised in the first five shots but the bullet was always there.

Safety-II approaches are prospective and a system is deemed safe if it can adjust to change within the system, that is, if it can demonstrate resilience. The focus is not on demonstrating causation of past incidents, but understanding the conditions that make things go right: what makes a system resilient.

Weick and Sutcliffe (2001) explored how industries including aircraft carriers, nuclear power plants and firefighting crews achieved reliably high performance. They found that the key for High Reliability Organisations (HROs) is in creating a state of system mindfulness that allows for the identification and correction of hazards before they are realised as adverse events. They described five principles that lead to mindfulness:

1 Preoccupation with failure
2 Reluctance to simplify interpretations
3 Sensitivity to operations
4 Commitment to resilience
5 Deference to expertise

There is a paucity of evidence about whether the principles and successes of HROs can be applied to healthcare but the increasing interest in exploring improvement approaches that respond to the changing dynamics of the system means it is starting to be considered. HROs are considered in detail in Chapter 7.

LEAN thinking

Chapter 1 introduced the 'LEAN' principles and these are now discussed further in the context of systems thinking. The term 'LEAN thinking' is a systems-based approach to quality management based on the production philosophy which evolved at Toyota, the car manufacturer in Japan. It is a philosophical approach to focusing on 'value': delivering the product or service with the minimum waste. The term was popularised by Womack et al. (1990) in their book *The Machine That Changed the World*, which described the thinking that had led to the dramatic difference in performance between Japanese car manufacturing and the rest of the world, and in particular the Toyota Production System (TPS). TPS sees operations as a unified flow, where each finished car represents a 'heartbeat', and the production process is one of pulling everything to that single end point. There are no intermediate points that are ends in themselves and everything else is considered in relation to its contribution to the finished car rolling off the production line. According to Seddon and Caulkin (2007):

> Where [TPS] saw flow and heartbeat, the Americans saw speed and volume. They saw that the faster they could 'push' work through the lines and the greater numbers of cars they made, the more cheaply and profitably they could do so. (p. 11)

The difference between pull and push reflects the difference between the focus of the system on a single output and the focus on completing individual tasks. The two pillars at Toyota were 'Just in Time' or flow of work and 'Jidoka' or intelligent automation. These two pillars were seen to dramatically reduce waste, both the unnecessary resources and the reduction in defective units. By considering the system as a whole and how different parts relate to each other, Toyota ensured that all actions were adding value to the system, and anything that was not active in adding some value was therefore waste and eliminated.

Previous production methods had managed work flow by developing standards and protocols for staff to follow but Toyota emphasised that this needed to be 'intelligent'. People should not unthinkingly follow the protocol but constantly consider whether the system is working well. Jidoka is about active thinking at the frontline, supported by protocols and standards rather than subsumed into them. For example, Toyota empowered its staff at all levels to 'Stop the line' even if that meant stopping the flow of the whole system.

LEAN is supported by a number of tools and techniques but remains primarily an approach that considers the physical and sociological systems that together deliver the product or service. LEAN has been applied to healthcare in which value is seen as a property of the system. That value is determined more by the design of the system than the will or expertise of individual members of staff. Berwick (2003) used the analogy that a car's top speed is limited by its design. No amount of incentives or sanctions will make it go faster and he draws comparison with the quality performance of healthcare systems, suggesting that there is a limit to improvements that can be made without redesigning the system.

Whilst LEAN is often discussed in relation to efficiency, Nelson-Peterson and Leppa (2007) described how the Virginia Mason Medical centre used LEAN thinking to create an environment for caring. They describe how the healthcare environment is often overburdened with non-value-added work that forms a barrier between the nurse and their ability to care for their patient. By reviewing and redesigning ward processes to focus on the system of the 'heartbeat' of the patient experience rather than intermediate tasks, they synchronised activities and improved communication, picked up changes in patients' status whilst reducing missed staff breaks. The changes have been accompanied by (rather than directed to) reductions in harms such as falls and pressure damage.

Microsystems

All systems are nested within larger systems and establishing the bounded areas of the systems is the first task for the improvement project leaders. The boundaries of a complex system are somewhat arbitrary and the default position has traditionally been an organisational structure but this may not be the most helpful definition for an improvement project. The system can be based on different parameters based on the nature of the improvement project. Some are based on patient pathways that make cross-organisational boundaries, whilst others are based on a process improvement within a single geographical location, on a uni-professional practice.

The smallest whole system is the microsystem, which is defined as a group of staff working together with a shared clinical purpose to provide care for a specified population of patients (Batalden and Splaine 2002). It can be argued that if individual microsystems are not delivering high quality, it will be impossible for the larger macro system to do so and therefore the microsystem is the most productive locale for quality improvement. By organising work around the smallest discrete, clinically focused system, the concept of a microsystem provides a window that illuminates the shared purpose within a single system and facilitates the integration of effort by people with different roles to deliver that common purpose. Once the microsystem boundaries have been defined and the staff develop a sense of shared social identity, the microsystem can develop focused task-based projects alongside developing the culture and the capability of the team for improvement. The focus of the clinical purpose of the microsystem rather than the organisational structure makes it an ideal model for engaging patients and clients as partners in improvement. A number of authors, including Nelson et al. (2011), have reported successful improvements using the microsystems approach and its use is growing. Box 3.2 shows how an English hospital used microsystem thinking to improve its paediatric service.

Box 3.2 A case study of how an English hospital used microsystem thinking to improve its paediatric service

Basildon and Thurrock University Hospitals NHS Foundation Trust had a four-bed paediatric assessment unit (PAU) co-located with the paediatric wards. The Care Quality Commission inspection in November 2012 reported significant failings within the service and the physical facilities. Closer working with the Children's Accident and Emergency Department (A and E) in the hospital was required to create one point of entry for all children and young people.

A multi-professional team reviewed the system and a decision was taken to move the PAU to the Accident and Emergency department. This allowed the team to create one front door access point for all unplanned paediatric attendances to the hospital; however, this provided challenges as the PAU service had to be redesigned to fit within the new location.

The number of children and young people coming through the A and E department increased with the move as all children with 'direct access' and direct referrals to paediatricians were not previously seen in A and E but now presented there and this put pressure on the existing children's A and E. All the additional children had to be triaged, additional equipment was needed and there were increases in medical consumables and drugs required in the department.

By January 2015, it was clear the move had improved the safety of children attending the hospital by having both the A and E and paediatric expertise in one area.

(*Continued*)

Box 3.2 A case study of how an English hospital used microsystem thinking to improve its paediatric service (*Continued*)

But the physical space was not sufficient and to be truly successful we needed additional space and to redesign the pathway for children attending the now termed Children's Emergency Department. To do this we approached it in the following way:

1   *We described our current operating system*
    As a team of Consultant Paediatrician, Paediatric Matron and Senior Children's A and E and PAU sisters, we mapped the patient journey from when the child arrived at the front door of A and E until the child left the department. This involved observing from the front door all the way through the department. Using Post-it notes, we identified and mapped every step of the patient journey.

2   *We evaluated this operating system*
    We needed to then identify what worked well in the process and what was waste in the process. Waste was determined as something that added no value to the patient or staff working in the department. This could be a repeated step in the process or was wasteful in terms of time or money.

3   *What does your patient value as important*
    We needed to meet with our children and young people and their families and ask them what they wanted from the service and what they valued as important when they attended the department. We identified families to engage with and we decided to approach families that had a chronic health need that had used the service since we moved. We also included families that had used the service and afterwards had raised an informal or formal complaint about their attendance.

    We asked the following questions:
    • What was important to them when they visited?
    • What could we do differently?
    • What did we do well?

    We asked families to be mystery shoppers for us, so that if they attended over the next 6 months could they provide feedback to us afterwards looking at the following questions:
    • Were staff welcoming and friendly?
    • Did they communicate clearly what was going to happen during the stay?
    • Were families asked if they were happy to take their child home?

4   *We looked at our staff and what was important to them*
    a) Did we have staff with the right skills? Are our teams comprised of the right mix of skills?
        • Are staff working to the top of their ability? Are staff doing tasks or making decisions for which they are overtrained? Undertrained?
        • Do staff have the authority to make the decisions and undertake the tasks they need to in the course of their work?

(Continued)

Box 3.2 A case study of how an English hospital used microsystem thinking to improve its paediatric service (*Continued*)

b) How do they feel about working in the department?
   - What do they value in working in the unit?
   - What non-value processes can they identify?
   - What suggestions do they have for working differently?

We then looked at all of our feedback and our processes and proposed a new operating model considering the following:

- Are key processes sufficiently standardised? Do we have a mechanism for dealing with nonstandard situations?
- Are processes as simple, linear and transparent as they can be?
- Have we removed unnecessary or non-value-adding steps from the key processes?
- Have we evaluated the risk (likelihood, potential impact) of potential failure of key processes and systems?

Development of a new system

Once we had answered all the questions, we worked together to develop a new operating model and we approached the estates team to design the new physical space for the PAU taking into account all the feedback of what worked and didn't work. A capital plan was designed for the new area.

In proposing a new model of care as a team, we took the decision that we could work differently in the new PAU by providing a short-stay facility for children and young people who required treatment and management of illnesses but were like to be able to be safely discharged home within 24 hours, and thereby we would be able to reduce the need for an acute inpatient admission.

Feedback from families was that they did not want to be admitted to the Paediatric inpatient ward if they did not need to be and that they would be happy to stay longer in the PAU, if that meant they would be discharged home sooner.

We identified five high-volume conditions that we felt could be safely managed within the PAU as a starting point; these all had associated care pathways for management. These were: fever, wheeze, gastroenteritis, bronchiolitis and head injury.

Implementation

The new short stay pathway to PAU was predicted to reduce the number of acute inpatient admissions to the wards and so we planned to reduce the number of inpatient beds from 24 to 20 beds. This allowed us to redeploy staff to the new short stay area by moving the 4.3 whole-time equivalent (WTE) of nursing staff via a 3- to 6-month rotation of staff. The medical team were already working in the department so this remained unchanged. Thus the new PAU required no additional funding for staff.

(*Continued*)

> **Box 3.2 A case study of how an English hospital used microsystem thinking to improve its paediatric service (*Continued*)**
>
> We also decided to review equipment such as multi-parameter monitors on the inpatient unit and move equipment to the PAU.
>
> Prior to opening the unit in September 2015, we invited the families that had been involved in the project back to see the new unit and explain the new pathway redesign and asked for feedback on the proposed new pathway. We then asked all families to physically go round the unit with post-it notes and give feedback on what was good and could be done differently. After the sessions we looked at the feedback and operational model to see whether any further improvements could be made.
>
> On the day we opened, the families were invited back in to see what changes we had made based on their feedback; changes were displayed in the form of a feedback board within the unit.
>
> During the first 4 weeks of opening, the senior team worked clinically on the unit to guide staff through the new pathway, answer questions, identify problems and provide support. As problems were identified, a Plan-Do-Study-Act (PDSA) cycle approach was taken to quickly identify an alternative way to work. Huddles were held five times a day when all nursing and medical staff came together to discuss all the PAU patients and management plans, safety issues identified, safeguarding concerns and any other concerns.

Integrating systems

Whilst the clinical microsystems approach works with co-located teams, many patients (especially those with multiple comorbidities) receive care from a number of discrete microsystems. Improving care for these people involves integrating systems. This may be integrating clinical teams from different specialities, integrating microsystems from different organisations and integrating health microsystems with social care microsystems.

As Shaw et al. (2011) noted, 'integrated care' is a term that reflects a desire to improve patient experience through better coordination and a combination of methods, processes and models. Integration is perceived to be a solution to the fragmentation of services leading to better continuity of care, more appropriate use of services and greater efficiency and value from health delivery. However, most of the literature discusses the perceived benefits rather than empirically observed outcomes of integration (Shaw et al. 2011).

In the United Kingdom, there has been a traditional lack of integrated services in health and social care but increasingly, from the late 1990s, health policies advocated better integration. The method of integration of systems is dependent on the intended objectives which will guide decisions about the processes that can best facilitate integrated care within any particular setting. Armitage et al.'s (2009) systematic review found three principal categories of integrations: vertical, horizontal and virtual:

- **Horizontal integration** focuses on organisations, networks or groups that appear to be providing similar care. This might include providing out-of-hospital services within a defined geographic area or integrating a medical speciality. Horizontal integration can provide higher levels of expertise across the working week by improved staff rotas and also economies of scale allowing wider access to technology.

- **Vertical integration** focuses on networks and groups at different stages of a patient's care journey within a specific health economy. This might lead to integration of primary and secondary services for a disease pathway but could also refer to the integration of all healthcare services within a geographical area, for example, the integration of acute hospitals, community and rehabilitation hospitals and community healthcare services (Baillie et al. 2014). Ham et al. (2011) argued that, due to demographic changes, the division between primary care and secondary care is increasingly unhelpful. Others have suggested that removing the traditional divide between hospital and community could resolve the reported communication issues between different healthcare providers at organisational level (Hanratty et al. 2012; Dossa et al. 2012).

- **Virtual integration** is an agreement to work collaboratively without the organisational change of a horizontal or vertical integration. At a regional level, cancer networks in the United Kingdom have been a highly effective form of virtual integration that has delivered significant quality improvement. At a local level, managing people with complex needs living in their own homes through virtual ward rounds that bring together a range of professionals both horizontally and vertically, has been shown to maintain independence and prevent hospital admission (see case study example, Box 3.3).

Box 3.3 Case study: Virtual wards

In a pilot scheme in the United Kingdom, virtual wards identified people who had a high risk of being admitted to hospital as an emergency intervention in the next 12 months. Virtual wards are a form of case management that promotes integration with social services and between primary and secondary care. The day-to-day work of the ward is led by a senior nurse who has prescribing and clinical examination skills with a virtual ward clerk, who acts as the central coordinator. The virtual ward staff include a named general practitioner, social workers and therapist. The team maintain close relationships with other organisations such as hospices and voluntary sector agencies and specialists from secondary care.

The virtual ward team share a common set of electronic notes and charts and conduct an office-based ward round each working day, with teleconference facilities available for staff who wish to join remotely. All newly admitted patients are discussed and existing patients are reviewed in turn and as required. All team members can suggest changes to the patient's care management plan and the team agree which staff member will perform which tasks.

Every night a list of each virtual ward's current patients is e-mailed securely to local hospitals and out-of-hours services. If any virtual ward patient arrives at an emergency department or calls an out-of-hours service, an alert that this patient belongs to a virtual ward is triggered. Secondary care staff can then contact the virtual ward clerk to obtain up-to-date information and work in partnership with the virtual ward staff to try to avoid a hospital admission or to arrange early discharge back to the care of the virtual ward team.

Source: Lewis, G., *Predictive Modelling In Action: How 'Virtual Wards' Help High-Risk Patients Receive Hospital Care at Home*, The Commonwealth Fund, New York, 2010.

Leutz (1999) described three different levels of integration: linkage, co-ordination and full integration:

1   **Linkage:** works best where people's needs are low intensity and ensures that staff from disparate systems have a core understanding of services available and referrals that can be made. There are no formal structures to link the systems.
2   **Co-ordination:** separate systems remain independent but some structures are put in place to align their work, usually in the form of joint appointment co-ordination managers.
3   **Full integration:** creates new structural units, where resources from the different systems are pooled and a new social identity and work processes are designed.

The most successful integration depends on the aims of the initiative and the degree of support from those most affected. Ramsay and Fulop (2008) suggest that top-down attempts (e.g., through mergers of service providers) are often less successful than those where the catalyst is the commitment of healthcare professionals for service improvement around a group of patients.

Integrated care initiatives tend to focus on either horizontal or vertical integration due to the structural challenges of achieving both simultaneously. Integration of two systems may result in the disintegration of a previous configuration and the unintended consequences as well as the benefits of integration should be considered. In addition, organisational integration alone will not lead to integrated working between professionals or improvements across the system (Baillie et al. 2014). Findings from a study of care transitions for frail older people within a vertically integrated healthcare system in England revealed that community and acute hospital staff lacked insight into services outside their own system, and there was a lack of trust among staff in different parts of the system too (Baillie et al. 2014). Thus, effective interprofessional working and collaboration are necessary to achieve integrated working in practice.

Interprofessional working and collaboration in practice

Interprofessional working is essential for ensuring coordinated and effective services for people accessing health and social care (Baillie and Black 2014) and arguably, services cannot be improved without effective interprofessional working either. In his 10 'top tips for scientific quality improvement', Goldmann (2011) advocated assembling a multi-professional team and ensuring that each have a clear and meaningful role. What is important then is that the team work collaboratively with patients, families and communities, because how well they work together affects patient care (Zwarenstein et al. 2009). The WHO (2010) defined collaborative practice as that which happens when:

> multiple health workers from different professional backgrounds work together with patients, families, carers and communities to deliver the highest quality of care.

> (WHO 2010, p. 7)

The WHO (2013) highlighted increasing interest internationally in the ability of healthcare professionals to work collaboratively together, identifying key enablers as the presence of leaders and champions, administrative and institutional support, mentorship and learning, shared vision and mission and an enabling built environment, that eliminates barriers to communication.

A survey of health and social care managers involved with care for older people in England revealed that the term 'interprofessional working' was not well recognised with people referring instead to working in partnership, integrated working or joint working depending on the sector within which they were based (Goodman et al. 2011). Nevertheless, there was support for the concept and there were plenty of examples offered, usually pathways related to a particular issue or condition, for example, falls prevention or stroke, and these involved working across organisations. Almost half of the respondents considered that professionals found it difficult to adapt to other professionals' ways of working and the majority considered there needed to be someone who took responsibility for ensuring the professionals worked effectively together, highlighting the importance of leadership. A review of the evidence for interprofessional teams in primary care, indicated that interprofessional models, including nurse-led teams, improved quality, patient satisfaction, access and equity (Jacobsen 2012). Interprofessional teams were considered cost-effective and advocated as the modality of choice in chronic disease management.

Collaboration is an interpersonal process that requires trust, mutual respect and effective communication (Colyer 2004; San Martin-Rodriguez et al. 2005) and there needs to be a regular dialogue among team members (Fabbre et al. 2011; Baillie et al. 2014). In a systematic review, Zwarenstein et al. (2009) found some evidence that practice-based initiatives to address interprofessional collaboration could have a positive effect on patient outcomes. As an example, Baillie et al. (2014) reported on how introducing daily facilitated multi-professional team meetings to review care transitions led to improved communication and relationships between the teams. This led on to streamlined processes so that organising family meetings became almost instantaneous rather than taking up to a week to organise.

Careau et al. (2015) developed a validated framework based on existing theory and stakeholder experience within rehabilitation for operationalising interprofessional collaboration in clinical settings. The final framework shows different types of practices according to four components: the situation of the client and family, the intention underlying the collaboration, the interaction between practitioners and the combining of disciplinary knowledge. Types of practices included:

- **Parallel practice**: Professionals encounter one or more other professionals in the course of working with patients and families but with minimal interaction.

- **Consultation/reference practice**: The exchange and sharing of information with at least one other professional with recognition of each other's roles but with still minimal interaction and mainly work in parallel (e.g., referrals).

- **Concerted practice**: Termed 'multidisciplinary' this involves planning and organising services based on the needs of the patient, family or community, with agreed objectives and coordination of services provided by multiple professionals.

- **Shared healthcare practice**: Termed 'interdisciplinary' this involves setting of common objectives and shared decision-making among the patient, family or community and the professionals.

They considered that the framework could enhance education about interprofessional collaboration as well as assisting practitioners and managers to optimise collaborative practice. Vachon et al. (2015) organised workshops with community professionals involved in the care of people with diabetes who identified improvement projects and plans for primary and or secondary prevention. They analysed the plans developing based on Careau et al.'s (2015) framework. Of the 22 plans developed, most involved consultation/reference practice or parallel practice with only two taking a concerted practice approach. Nevertheless, the authors concluded that the interprofessional approach for planning quality improvement was a successful approach, though it clearly needed further development.

The Canadian Interprofessional Health Collaborative identified the following six competency domains for effective working of interprofessional collaborative practice: (1) patient/client/family/community-centred care, (2) communication, (3) collaborative teamwork, (4) conflict resolution, (5) role clarification and (6) collaborative leadership (Hepp et al. 2015). An analysis of qualitative data from six acute care units revealed good practice in most domains, but there needed to be better role clarification and collaborative leadership in interprofessional rounds needed improving too. A common source of conflict was around discharge planning. Use of this framework assisted in identifying areas for improvement.

Interprofessional collaboration in quality improvement

It is hard to think of any area of healthcare practice where one professional group works alone and therefore a starting point for any improvement project idea is to identify all the professional groups involved within the specific microsystem and other linked microsystems, including both clinical and non-clinical services. You also need to plan how patients, families and communities can be involved from the start of the improvement work as part of the collaborating team (see Box 3.2 for an example and Chapter 4).

There are a number of published examples of interprofessional working in quality improvement. For example, Engel et al. (2013) reported on an interprofessional quality improvement project to implement an intensive care unit early mobility programme, which involved nursing, physiotherapy and physicians and led to positive outcomes: reduced intensive care unit and hospital length of stay and decreased rates of delirium and the need for sedation for the patients. As another example, based on an oncology ward, Bohnenkamp et al. (2014a, b) reported on an interprofessional quality improvement project to reduce venothromboembolism through increased compliance with an evidence-based intervention: the sequential compression device. At the project start, compliance with the compression device was 59%, which was increased to 100% through applying three Plan-Do-Study-Act (PDSA) cycles. The staff worked collaboratively with patients and families as to the best educational approach to use. The professionals involved included nurses (ward-based, infection control, clinical nurse specialists), physicians, purchasing staff and housekeeping, highlighting the importance of non-clinical staff members and departments in quality improvement initiatives. Box 3.4 details

Box 3.4 Interprofessional working in quality improvement

There is evidence that immediate skin-to-skin contact (SSC) between mother and infant increases breastfeeding success but traditionally, SSC may not be instigated for women who undergo a caesarean section until after they leave the operating theatre. Brady et al. (2014) reported on an interprofessional quality improvement project in the United States, which led to more women/infant SSC during caesarean sections and increased breastfeeding rates. This was a complex change involving a range of disciplines working within different though linked microsystems: the operating theatre and pre-natal care. The project also involved a change to the electronic medical record (to record that

(Continued)

Box 3.4 Interprofessional working in quality improvement (*Continued*)

the woman had been educated about SSC and agreed) and the introduction of a new nursing role to support SSC in the operating theatre.

The interprofessional team members were identified as the women themselves, nurses, breastfeeding coordinators, scrub technicians, obstetricians, anaesthetists, neonatologists, paediatricians and lactation consultants. During planning, the concerns of the different disciplines were revealed: nurses were concerned that the infant would get cold and that the mother would not be able to hold the infant well enough, obstetricians were concerned that the baby's feet might slip under the drape and compromise asepsis, anaesthetists were concerned they might be responsible for monitoring the infant as well as the mother and paediatricians were concerned about the nurses' ability to monitor the newborn infant during the SSC. It was also identified that some mothers might feel embarrassed to expose their breasts in the operating theatre or they may not be physiologically stable enough. Educational needs for all professionals and the mothers were identified and planned.

In the first PDSA cycle, the SSC was tried successfully with two mothers who gave positive feedback. In subsequent PDSA cycles, any barriers continued to be identified and addressed and nurse champions for SSC acted as peer coaches; gradually more staff engaged with the changed practice. The progress of SSC was disseminated across the interprofessional team. After 6 months, SSC was fully established in the operating theatre. Exclusive breastfeeding rates of women undergoing caesarean section increased from 8% to 19% in the same period.

a further example and is also a good illustration of the involvement of two microsystems (pre-natal care and the operating theatre) in a quality improvement initiative.

Conclusion

This chapter has explained systems thinking and how this relates to healthcare and improvement. As healthcare has become increasingly complex, in order to respond to a population who often have multiple health needs resulting from long-term conditions, improvement activity cannot be carried out in isolation but must be a collaborative activity with other healthcare professionals, patients, families and communities. Healthcare can be thought of as multiple microsystems within larger systems and any planning for improvement must start by considering what constitutes the system, and what other microsystems must be included in the improvement work too. This chapter explored different ways of integrating services as these could better enable improvement work. Effective collaborative interprofessional working is essential for improving quality, as illustrated in this chapter's case study examples.

References

Armitage, G.D., Suter, E., Oelke, N.D., and Adair, C.E. (2009) Health systems integration: State of the evidence. *International Journal of Integrated Care* 9(2): e82.

Baillie, L. and Black, S. (2014) *Professional Values in Nursing*. Boca Raton, FL: Taylor & Francis.

Baillie, L., Gallini, A., Corser, R., Elsworthy, G., Leeder, A., and Barrand, A. (2014) Care transitions for frail, older people from acute hospital wards within an integrated healthcare system in England: A qualitative case study. *International Journal of Integrated Care* 14(1): e009.

Batalden, P. and Splaine, M. (2002) What will it take to lead the continual improvement and innovation of health care in the twenty-first century? *Quality Management in Healthcare* 11(1): 45–54.

Berwick, D. (2003) Improvement, trust, and the healthcare workforce. *Quality and Safety in Health Care* 12: i2–i6.

Bohnenkamp, S., Pelton, N., Rishel, C.J., and Kurtin, S. (2014a) Implementing evidence-based practice: Using an interprofessional team approach. *Oncology Nursing Forum* 41(4): 434–437.

Bohnenkamp, S., Pelton, N., Rishel, C.J., and Kurtin, S. (2014b) Implementing evidence-based practice: Using an interprofessional team approach. Part 2. *Oncology Nursing Forum* 41(5): 548–550.

Brady, K., Bulpitt, D., and Chiarelli, C. (2014) An interprofessional quality improvement project to implement maternal/infant skin-to-skin contact during caesarean section. *Journal of Obstetric, Gynecologic, and Neonatal Nursing* 43: 488–496.

Careau, E., Brière, N., Houle, N., Dumont, S., Vincent, C., and Swaine, B. (2015) Interprofessional collaboration: Development of a tool to enhance knowledge translation. *Disability and Rehabilitation* 37(4):372–378.

Checkland, P. (1999) *Systems Thinking, Systems Practice; Soft Systems Methodology: A 30-Year Retrospective*. Chichester: John Wiley & Sons.

Colyer, H.M. (2004) The construction and development of health professions: Where will it end? *Journal of Advanced Nursing* 48(4): 406–412.

Dekker, S. (2007) Doctors are more dangerous than gun owners: A rejoinder to error counting. *Human Factors* 49(20): 177–184.

Deming, W.E (1993) *The New Economics for Industry, Government, and Education*. Boston, MA: MIT Press.

Dossa, A., Bokhour, B., and Hoenig, H. (2012) Care transitions from the hospital to home for patients with mobility impairments: Patient and family caregiver experiences. *Rehabilitation Nursing* 37(6): 277–285.

Engel, H.J., Needham, D.M., Morris, P.E., and Gropper, M.A. (2013) ICU early mobilization: From recommendation to implementation at three medical centers. *Critical Care Medicine* Supplement. 41: S69–80.

Fabbre, V.D., Buffington, A.S., Altfeld, S.J., Shier, G.E., and Golden, R.L. (2011) Social work and transitions of care: Observations from an intervention for older adults. *Journal of Gerontological Social Work* 54(6): 615–626.

Forrester, J. (1971) Counterintuitive behavior of social systems. *Technology Review* 73(3): 52–68.

Goldmann, D. (2011) Ten tips for incorporating scientific quality improvement into everyday work. *BMJ Quality and Safety* 20(1): i69–i72.

Goodman, C., Drennan, V., Scheibl, F., Shah, D., Manthorpe, J., Gage, H., and Iliffe, S. (2011) Models of inter professional working for older people living at home: A survey and review of the local strategies of English health and social care statutory organisations. *BMC Health Services Research* 14(11): 337.

Ham, C., Imison, C., Goodwin, N., Dixon, A., and South, P. (2011) *Where Next for the NHS Reforms? The Case for Integrated Care*. London: King's Fund.

Hanratty, B., Holmes, L., Lowson, E., Grande, G., Addington-Hall, J., Payne, S., et al. (2012) Older adults' experiences of transitions between care settings at the end of life in England: A qualitative interview study. *Journal of Pain and Symptom Management* 44(1): 74–83.

Haynes, A.B., Weiser, T.G., Berry, W.R., Lipsitz, S.R., Breizat, A.H., Dellinger, E.P., et al. (2011) Changes in safety attitude and relationship to decreased postoperative morbidity and mortality following implementation of a checklist-based surgical safety intervention. *BMJ Quality and Safety* 20(1): 102–107.

Hepp, S.L., Suter, E., Jackson, K., Deutschlander, S., Makwarimba, E., Jennings, J., and Birmingham, L. (2015) Using an interprofessional competency framework to examine collaborative practice. *Journal of Interprofessional Care* 29(2):131–137.

Hollnagel, E., Braithwaite, J., and Wears, R.L., editors (2013) *Resilient Health Care*. Farnham, UK: Ashgate Publishing, Ltd.

Jacobsen, P.M. (2012) *Evidence Synthesis for Interprofessional Teams in Primary Care*. Commissioned paper for the Canadian Nurses' Association. Canadian Health Services Research Foundation. Available from: www.chsrf.ca (accessed on 25 September 2016).

Lewis, G. (2010) *Predictive Modelling in Action: How 'Virtual Wards' Help High-Risk Patients Receive Hospital Care at Home*. New York, NY: The Commonwealth Fund.

Leutz, W.N. (1999) Five laws for integrating medical and social services: Lessons from the United States and the United Kingdom. *Milbank Quarterly* 77(1): 77–110.

Nelson, E.C., Batalden, P.B. and Godfrey, M.M., editors. (2011) *Quality by Design: A Clinical Microsystems Approach*. Hoboken, NJ: John Wiley & Sons.

Nelson-Peterson, D.L. and Leppa, C.J. (2007) Creating an environment for caring using lean principles of the Virginia Mason Production System. *Journal of Nursing Administration* 37(6): 287–294.

Pickering, S., Robertson, E.R., and Griffin, D. (2013) Compliance and use of the World Health Organization checklist in UK operating theatres. *British Journal of Surgery* 100(12): 1664–1670.

Ramsay, A. and Fulop, N. (2008) *The Evidence Base for Integrated Care*. London: Department of Health.

Reason, J. (1997) *Managing the Risks of Organizational Accidents*. Aldershot: Ashgate.

Seddon, J. and Caulkin, S. (2007) Systems thinking, lean production and action learning. *Action Learning: Research and Practice* 4(1): 9–24.

Senge, P.M. (1990) *The Fifth Discipline*. New York, NY: Currency Doubleday.

Schein, E.H. (2013) *Humble Inquiry: The Gentle Art of Asking Instead of Telling*. San Francisco, CA: Berrett-Koehler Publishers.

Shaw, S., Rosen, R., and Rumbold, B. (2011) *What Is Integrated Care?* London: Nuffield Trust.

San Martin-Rodriguez, L., Beaulieu, M.D., D'Amour, D., and Ferrada-Videla, M. (2005) The determinants of successful collaboration: A review of theoretical and empirical studies. *Journal of Interprofessional Care* 19(Suppl. 1): 132–147.

Vachon, B., Désorcy, B., Gaboury, I., Camirand, M., Rodrigue, J., Quesnel, L., Guimond, C., Labelle, M., Huynh, A.T., and Grimshaw, J. (2015) Combining administrative data feedback, reflection and action planning to engage primary care professionals in quality improvement: Qualitative assessment of short term program outcomes. *BMC Health Services Research* 18(15): 391.

van Klei, W.A., Hoff, R.G., van Aarnhem, E.E.H.L., Simmermacher, R.K.J., Regli, L.P.E., Kappen, T.H., van Wolfswinkel, L., Kalkman, C.J., Buhre, W.F., Peelen, L.M. (2012) Effects of the introduction of the WHO "Surgical Safety Checklist" on in-hospital mortality: A cohort study. *Annals of Surgery* 255(1): 44–49.

Vincent, C., Taylor-Adams, S., Chapman, E., and Hewett, D. (2000) How to investigate and analyse clinical incidents: Clinical risk unit and association of litigation and risk management protocol. *British Medical Journal* 320(7237): 777.

Vincent, C., and Amalberti, R. (2016) *Safer Healthcare*. Switzerland: Springer International Publishing.

Von Bertalanffy, L. (1968) *General Systems Theory: Foundations, Development, Applications*. New York, NY: Braziller.

Weick, K. and Sutcliffe, K. (2001) *Managing the Unexpected: Assuring High Performance in an Age of Complexity*. San Francisco: Jossey-Bass.

Womack, J.P., Jones, T.D., and Roos, D. (1990) *The Machine That Changed the World*. New York, NY: Free Press.

World Health Organisation (2010) *Framework for Action on Interprofessional Education and Collaborative Practice*. Switzerland: World Health Organization. Available from: http://whqlibdoc.who.int/hq/2010/WHO_HRH_HPN_10.3_eng.pdf (accessed on 25 September 2016).

World Health Organisation (2013) *Interprofessional Collaborative Practice in Primary Healthcare: Nursing and Midwifery Perspectives. Six Case Studies*. Geneva: World Health Organisation. Available from: http://www.who.int/hrh/resources/IPE_SixCaseStudies.pdf (accessed on 25 September 2016).

Zwarenstein, M., Goldman, J., and Reeves, S. (2009) Interprofessional collaboration: Effects of practice-based interventions on professional practice and healthcare outcomes. *Cochrane Database Systematic Reviews* 8(3). Available from: http://onlinelibrary.wiley.com/doi/10.1002/14651858.CD000072.pub2/full (accessed on 25 September 2016).

4 Service User Involvement in Healthcare Improvement

Nicola Thomas

Introduction

Service user involvement in improvement work continues to develop, yet to date, efforts have not necessarily focused on the patients' experience beyond asking what was good and what was not (Bate and Robert 2006). This chapter discusses the innovative ways in which service and quality improvement (QI) projects can involve service users in their design and delivery. The chapter also provides practical case studies of service user involvement.

'Service user' is used here as an umbrella term to include people who have health conditions, people who are caregivers (including carers, parents and family members) and others with relevant lived experience (such as those who have experience of social care).

Objectives

The chapter's objectives are to:

- Identify how service user involvement in QI has evolved over recent years
- Discuss the ways in which service and QI projects can successfully involve service users in their design and delivery
- Analyse how service user involvement in service and QI can be evaluated
- Provide practical examples of service user involvement that can be replicated in other contexts
- Explore the possible ways in which impact of service user involvement in QI can be assessed

Introduction to service user involvement in healthcare

Policy and practice background

The 'National Health Service (NHS) and Community Care Act' (1990) has been widely cited as the first piece of UK legislation to establish a formal requirement for service user involvement in healthcare planning and improvement. This was closely followed by the Patient's Charter (1991) which emphasised the UK government's intention to provide 'patient-centred' care and ensure that the patient's voice was heard. Ten years later, the Health and Social Care Act (2001a) required all NHS trusts, primary care trusts (PCTs) and strategic health authorities to consult with and involve people in service planning and evaluation. The Act stated that:

It is the duty ... that persons to whom those services are being or may be provided for, are directly or through representatives, involved in and consulted on:

a) the planning of the provision of those services,
b) the development and consideration of proposals for changes in the way those services are provided, and
c) decisions to be made by that body affecting the operation of those services.

(Department of Health [DH] 2001, p. 11)

'*Involving Patients and the Public in Health Care*' (DH 2001b) developed mechanisms for putting into place the legislation of the Health and Social Care Act (DH 2001a). This included a programme for setting up patient forums in every PCT and NHS Trust, the setting up of a Commission for Patient and Public Involvement in Health and requiring every NHS trust and PCT to publish an account of how the public had been involved in services. In 2008, the Care Quality Commission (CQC) became the regulator of all health and adult social care services and was required by government to promote awareness among service users of its functions, engage with service users about the provision of health and social care services and ensure that the views of service users are respected.

Two years later, the principle of 'no decision about me, without me' was highlighted in the white paper *Equity and Excellence: Liberating the NHS* (DH, 2010). The white paper identified that information generated by patients themselves will be critical to this ideology and will include much wider use of effective tools like Patient-Reported Outcome Measures (PROMS), patient experience data and real-time feedback (DH 2010, p. 14).

In 2014, England's health authorities were abolished and funds transferred to new general practitioner (GP)-led clinical commissioning groups (CCGs). The CCGs have a legal duty to promote the involvement of service users and their carers or representatives in decisions that relate to the prevention or diagnosis of illness or in their care or treatment. In addition, health and wellbeing boards have been established, although there has been some uncertainty and confusion with regard to service user involvement in the new structures such as the different perspectives users and professionals may have on the impact of user involvement in commissioning, and demands that are placed on single service user representatives, that is, the time necessary for meaningful involvement (Evans et al. 2015).

More recently, an inquiry was undertaken into the serious failings of the Mid Staffordshire NHS Foundation Trust in England between 2005 and 2008. The report (Francis 2013) called for a fundamental culture shift within the NHS and emphasised the need for patient-centred care and involvement. The report stated that the management at the trust did not have a culture of listening to patients and asking for feedback. One of the consequences was that the UK policy was amended to reflect these criticisms and the NHS Constitution, updated in 2015, has stated that 'The NHS will actively encourage feedback from the public, patients and staff, welcome it and use it to improve its services' (DH 2015).

Involving service users in improvement projects – Where are we now?

Although recent policy initiatives highlighted in England have seen an increased emphasis on service user involvement in QI over the past decade, meaningful involvement by service users faces continuing challenges. It is possible that although hospitals have attempted to engage patients in QI, some attempts, such as patient surveys, have been used as 'tick box' exercises with patients never seeing whether their suggestions have been acted upon. Also patient-experience data, often presented to hospital boards, are 'noted for information' rather than leading to action points and organisational learning (Dr Foster Intelligence 2010).

Despite organisations such as the Health Foundation in the United Kingdom and the Institute for Health Improvement in the United States, making numerous recommendations and providing resources to enable involvement, some clinicians find it difficult to understand *whether* and *how* service users can be involved in improvement projects in significant and distinctive ways (Armstrong et al. 2013).

Another challenge is *who* exactly should be involved in QI. As Armstrong et al. (2013) have discussed, there is often debate on whether service users should be representative of the demographic characteristics of the population from which they are drawn or whether it is preferable that they represent shared experiences and standpoints and have particular kinds of skills and capacities (Martin 2008).

Co-production of service and QI projects

Evidence-based co-design

Design-led professions, such as architecture and computer graphics have long held the common aim that a product or process should be as user-friendly as possible and within the health service new ways that enable patients and staff to design and improve services are emerging (Tollyfield 2014). As an example, a model for evidence-based co-design (EBCD), originally developed by Bate and Robert (2007), has been used to develop services in a number of specialities, including cancer care (Tsianakas et al. 2012) and critical care (Tollyfield 2014), with projects typically taking 6–12 months to complete.

EBCD is an approach to improving healthcare services that combines participatory and user experience design tools and processes to bring about QIs in healthcare organisations. Through a 'co-design' process, the approach involves staff, patients and carers reflecting on their experiences of a service, working together to identify improvement priorities, devising and implementing changes and then jointly reflecting on their achievements (Bate and Robert 2007).

As the authors described,

> In its complete sense, users may be involved in every step of the design process from diagnosis and need analysis, through envisioning and model building, to prototyping and testing, implementing and evaluating. And in this process they do not just say things, they do things as well; and they do them in person, not through some third party.
>
> (Bate and Robert 2007, p. 30)

This approach commences with an exploratory phase where service users are interviewed and observations of the environment made. Resulting themes from the interviews and observations are identified, and later, staff and patients come together to discuss the themes that emerged from the interviews. However, some authors have suggested that although the EBCD approach exemplifies the unique contribution that service users can make in *identifying* problems of quality and safety in healthcare, it is less clear how service users can contribute to *improving* processes and quality of care (Entwistle et al. 2010).

Step-by-step guide to involving service users in improvement work

Although there is a growing emphasis for inclusion of the patient's voice in improvement of healthcare quality, there continues to be few published papers on practical ways to involve service users in improvement work. This chapter presents an easy-to-follow, step-by-step guide to involving service users in improvement work, based on recommendations from a research team that evaluated three very different models of patient involvement via an ethnographic approach involving 126 in-depth interviews, 12 weeks of non-participant observations and documentary analysis of three QI projects (Armstrong et al., 2013).

The three projects differed in the ways they involved patients, acting in some cases as intermediaries between the wider patient community and clinicians and sometimes undertaking persuasive work to convince clinicians of the need for change. The team then identified specific strategies that can be used to help ensure that patient involvement works most effectively (Armstrong et al. 2013): see Box 4.1.

Ensure clarity on the rationale for patient involvement

Prior to the start of any improvement work, it is important that the improvement team takes time to think through the rationale for involving service users. First, the focus of the involvement needs to be clarified: is it to *identify and prioritise* needs or resources, to *monitor and evaluate* services or to *improve services* using a recognised QI methodology? In addition, the team needs to consider the ways in which service users are representative: to contribute their *own* voice or experience or to contribute the voice of a *group* of people with a specific condition for example. An unclear rationale and focus for the involvement at the first stage can easily slip into tokenism (Armstrong et al. 2013).

Attention needs to be paid to the way in which service users are recruited, as it is often common to involve service users who are well known within community or self-help groups. One effective way to do this is to enroll one service user who is already well known to clinicians and also within the patient/carer population and then ask them to recruit others. It is crucial to actively seek people who are traditionally 'hard to reach', especially if they are representative of the population that is being served. Good practice is to monitor who is being involved in QI, so that gaps in representation are identified and seldom heard groups are targeted where appropriate.

Suitable ways to engage service users in QI include:

- Advertising in waiting areas of outpatient departments and GP practices: giving postcards out at reception to people who are booking in is often much more successful as a way of recruiting than a poster on a noticeboard

---

Box 4.1 Recommendations for successful service user involvement in quality improvement

- Ensure clarity on the rationale for patient involvement.
- Identify the appropriate involvement model to achieve the desired outcomes.
- Discuss and provide clear roles and responsibilities for service users.
- Ensure involvement is meaningful (and measure the effects of the involvement).

Source: Adapted from Armstrong, N. et al., *Health Expect.*, 16(3), e36–e47, 2013.

- Advertising in newsletters (self-help groups, leisure groups, libraries)
- Making direct contact with self-help groups, such as Expert Patient Programmes or local Healthwatch organisations
- Clinical staff making an approach to individual patients directly

Identify the appropriate involvement model to achieve the desired outcomes

Armstrong et al. (2013) suggested that issues such as the nature of the quality gap, the clinical area, the improvement tools being used and the characteristics of the patients served should be considered next. There are many different ways in which people might participate in improvement depending upon their personal circumstances and interest. The 'Ladder of Engagement and Participation' (Arnstein 1969) is a widely recognised model for understanding different forms and degrees of patient and public involvement. Figure 4.1 (adapted from Arnstein) shows one way in which practitioners can evaluate their involvement practices: by asking themselves where on the ladder they believe their interactions with future service users are located. In QI, it is important that both clinicians and service users have the same expectations of their involvement and if there is conflict then service users may feel disempowered and disheartened. Finally, be flexible about the role patients can play and tailor to the project's context.

Discuss and provide clear roles and responsibilities for service users

It is extremely important to discuss the roles and responsibilities of service users prior to them having any involvement in QI. Good practice includes the writing of a role description that can be used when advertising for service users to be involved. Box 4.2 shows the items that need to be considered when writing a role description, although it is important that service users develop the scope of the role themselves where appropriate.

Service users can undertake a variety of roles and at the start of the QI project it is important to spend time discussing prior knowledge and skills and also learning needs. It is also important to give constructive feedback on their involvement, just the same as for other colleagues. Service users and carers have unique skills and abilities and are 'experts' in their own illness and experts by experience. In addition to these skills and experiences, clinicians should actively seek service users' other skills, such as information technology, marketing, commissioning and so on. Training in both QI and other skills, such as teaching, need to be provided to build confidence and allow full participation.

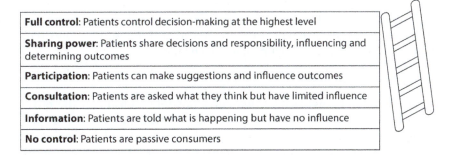

Figure 4.1 The engagement ladder. (Adapted from Arnstein, S., *J. Am. Plann. Assoc.*, 35(4), 216–224, 1969.)

Box 4.2 Items to be considered when writing a role description for service users involved in quality improvement (QI) projects

Information about the QI project

Responsibilities of role

Approximate time the involvement work will take per week

- Regular communication by e-mail/letter etc. – how often
- Reading of relevant paperwork prior to meetings
- Attendance at meetings – frequency, where, when
- Other activities, for example writing the project proposal, being involved in securing funds to undertake the project, writing of letters to gain support from other service users, writing of patient stories, development of patient education materials, spreading the successes of the QI project

Payment

Expenses and if payment for the service user's time, how to claim and the method of payment. The guidance from INVOLVE is helpful (see Section "Useful Resources" at the end of the chapter)

Other benefits

Training on QI, development of presentation skills and conference attendance

Feedback

Whether there is a process for giving feedback on performance

Confidentiality when working on the project

Main point of contact and what to do if unwell/unable to commit to role

Remuneration for involvement requires particular attention, and this needs to be discussed carefully with the service user at the outset. The service user may decide not to claim payment for their time, as this may impact on any benefits they receive. The QI team should also ensure that relevant tax and employment laws are complied with. An easy process to claim remuneration should be put in place and all expenses should be paid promptly. The DH's (2006) Reward and Recognition Policy is now outdated, but there are helpful recommendations within the policy that recognise the different levels of input and expertise required by service users for different activities, and that different but consistent reward is offered according to the level at which people are engaging.

Ensure involvement is meaningful

It is crucial to ensure early involvement wherever possible – ideally at the protocol-design stage. Effective communication within the team is also critical and discussion about the most effective methods of communication is required. For example, plain English, large print, braille, British Sign Language and minority languages might all need to be considered. Also, it is important not to assume that all service users have access to e-mail or the Internet, so alternatives may be required.

Clinicians need to pay attention to creating a non-hierarchical structure, especially in meetings, by valuing and giving weight to each team member's views. The case study (see Box 4.3) highlights the differing roles that patients and carers can have within QI teams.

Box 4.3 Case study: Service user involvement in quality improvement (QI)

The overall aim of the ASSIST-CKD project (running from 2015–2018) is early identification of people with declining kidney function through laboratory-based graphical surveillance of long-term trends in kidney function. Kidney Research UK is leading this UK-wide project, supported by the Health Foundation, and the project involves 20 renal units, pathology laboratories, their surrounding GP practices and CCGs. In the laboratories, a graph of kidney function over time is generated for patients with reduced kidney function (estimated glomerular filtration rate [eGFR]). The graph is then reviewed by a trained member of the laboratory team (or renal nurse). For patients showing a declining eGFR trajectory, the graph and a report highlighting the trend, is sent to the GP.

There is active involvement of patients in the ASSIST-CKD project via the Patient Project Team (PPT). Members of the PPT not only have personal experience of kidney disease and its impact but also bring their wider commercial expertise to support the project. Two members of the PPT were late-referred to secondary care (defined as referred less than 3 months before requiring dialysis) and therefore know only too well the additional challenges this brings to their patient journey. All members of the PPT are keen to tell their own stories and share their experiences.

> … if my GP had diagnosed me earlier, I could have made small lifestyle changes and taken medication which could have slowed the progression into kidney failure.

One member of the PPT was on dialysis for over 23 years before receiving a living-related kidney donation in May 2011. Now retired, he was previously a career banker responsible for setting up and leading the Islamic Financial Services Division in the United Kingdom for a major UK bank. He played an integral part of putting together the business case for the project, which will be used by renal units in support of seeking ongoing funding from CCGs to sustain the project. He was able to use his unique insight and experience to help produce an infographic, which supported the business case.

Another patient, who has also received a kidney transplant, has been involved in communicating with key contacts within local kidney patient associations and the renal unit's media teams. He has also described his personal kidney journey to a project learning event, which was effective in communicating how the project's intervention can have a positive impact for patients.

Another member of the PPT is a locum GP and she has also experienced long-term dialysis. She has been able to give practical and effective guidance as a voice of primary care – what happens on a day-to-day basis in GP surgeries and how this can impact the success of the project. Other members of the PPT have attended conferences on behalf of the project team, for example, attendance at an NHS Preventative Health event, where it was aimed to promote the important message about CKD as part of the NHS Healthcheck programme.

For further information, visit https://www.kidneyresearchuk.org/research/assist-ckd.

Evaluation of service user involvement in QI

Trier et al. (2015) reviewed research published between 2006 and 2011 concerning the involvement of patients in patient safety initiatives in primary care. The authors however found only weak evidence that supported a positive impact of patient involvement on improving patient safety and suggested that barriers to successful involvement included patient characteristics and the attitudes of health professionals. It could however be questioned whether the outcome measures used to measure impact were appropriate or indeed whether outcome measures were comparable across all studies, making comparison difficult.

Boaz et al. (2016) explored the different roles adopted by 63 patients within four participatory QI interventions and measured the nature of their impact upon implementation processes and outcomes. Two key themes emerged from the data. First, the authors found a range of different roles adopted by patients within and across the four projects; these ranged from sharing of experiences, through to involvement in developing potential solutions and implementing those solutions. Some people became 'experts by experience' through engaging in the whole co-design process. Second, patients and carers acted as catalysts for broader change in the attitudes of staff by providing a motivation for wider organisational and attitudinal changes.

Despite little evidence to suggest that there are real benefits in involving patients in QI, it is crucial that QI team members reflect on how well they involved people in the QI process. Box 4.4 identifies suitable questions to ask during evaluation.

Capturing the patient experience

The 1000 Lives Plus initiative from NHS Wales, defined the term 'patient stories' as the experience of a range of potential storytellers, communicating for different reasons with a range of different audiences. For example, the story can be from a patient or family member who has experienced excellent care or improvement in services or a story can be from someone who has had an unsatisfactory experience of healthcare. Patient stories have gained acceptance as engagement strategies in QI and might be used as a starting point as a QI project rationale. There is often however, little clarity about how to use patient stories and they could risk becoming a token response to the patient involvement agenda.

The main aim is to gain an understanding of the healthcare experience of the storyteller: what was good, what was bad and what would make the experience more positive. Patient stories have unique features which make them appropriate in QI projects. An outline of these features is shown in Figure 4.2.

Box 4.5 presents a case study that will help you to understand how to use patient narratives to improve quality and also improve efficiency, in an outpatient setting.

Box 4.4 Evaluation of service user involvement in quality improvement (QI)

- At what point in the QI process were service users involved?
- What methods were used to engage patients in QI, and why were they chosen?
- Was participation encouraged and made easy?
- What methods were used to really listen to patients?

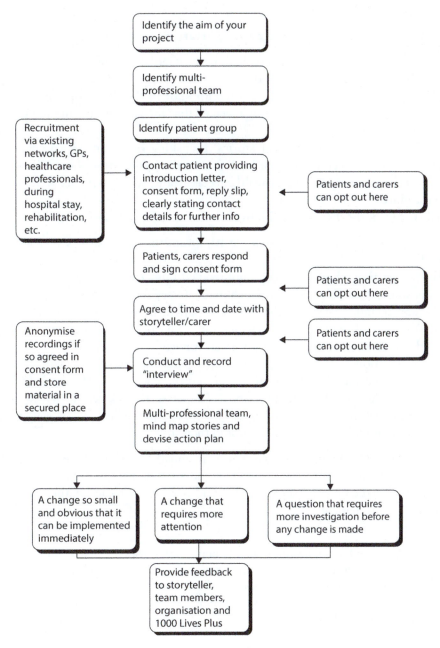

Figure 4.2 Strategies for the collection and use of patient stories. (From NHS Wales, 2011, *Learning to Use Patient Stories*, available from: http://www.1000livesplus.wales.nhs.uk/. With permission.)

Conclusion

This chapter has discussed the background to service user involvement in healthcare and the ways in which service users can be fully involved in improvement work. Practical tips and resources to support involvement in a meaningful way have been presented. It is important to reflect on how service user involvement in QI can be evaluated in the future, because,

Box 4.5 Case study: Using service user narratives in improvement

An endoscopy unit was experiencing a high percentage of patients who could not have their flexible colonoscopy as planned because of poor pre-endoscopy bowel preparation. This resulted in inefficient use of time for staff in the endoscopy unit. Informal discussion with patients pre-endoscopy revealed that the patient information sheet was not clear.

It was decided to collect 'patient stories' by asking each patient who arrived for endoscopy over a 1-week period, for feedback on the information sheet. The informal discussions were undertaken by a healthcare assistant, whilst patients were awaiting their procedure.

Feedback from the discussions discovered that

- The information sheet's font size (size 10) meant that the text was very difficult to read.
- The information sheet had been photocopied numerous times by the admissions team, so there was blurred text which made it very difficult to read.
- The text included language that was not patient-friendly. For example, the term OGD was used, without any explanation. Some people did not understand the word 'medication' and did not realise that it meant an enema.
- The instructions for diet and clear fluids made no sense. The letter said that patients could have a light breakfast before the enema and then should use the enema 1–2 hours before the procedure. The letter also suggested that the patient could 'have clear fluids up to 2 hours before the procedure' but it was not clear whether that meant that all fluids should then stop.

As a result of the findings, the letter was amended in collaboration with patients. Procedures were put in place to ensure that the admissions unit always had an electronic version of the updated sheet on file and knew where to access the updated version to send out to patients.

although health policy has suggested that it is beneficial, strong evidence is required to support the assertion that meaningful involvement makes a difference to health and social care. Finally, the capturing of patient narratives and their contribution to QI has been explained. There are a growing number of useful resources for service user involvement and these are recommended further reading.

Useful resources

Health Foundation. Involving Patients in Improving Safety. http://www.health.org.uk/publication/involving-patients-improving-safety

Healthwatch. http://www.healthwatch.co.uk/

Institute for Health Improvement. Engaging Patients and Families as Partners. http://www.ihi.org/resources/Pages/ImprovementStories/DeliveringGreatCareEngagingPatientsandFamiliesasPartners.aspx.

INVOLVE Reward and Recognition. http://www.invo.org.uk/wp-content/uploads/2012/09/INVOLVE PaymentGuiderev2012.pdf

Kings College London: Experience-Based Co-Design (EBCD). http://www.kingsfund.org.uk/projects/ebc

References

Armstrong, N., Herbert, G., Aveling, E.-L., Dixon-Woods, M., and Martin, G. (2013) Optimizing patient involvement in quality improvement. *Health Expectations* 16(3): e36–e47.

Arnstein, S. (1969) A ladder of citizen participation. *Journal of the American Planning Association* 35(4): 216–224.

Bate, P. and Robert, G. (2006) Experience-based design: From redesigning the system around the patient to co-designing services with the patient. *Quality and Safety in Health Care* 15(5): 307–310.

Bate, P. and Robert, G. (2007) *Bringing User Experience to Healthcare Improvement: The Concepts, Methods and Practices of Experience-Based Design*. Oxford: Radcliffe Publishing.

Boaz, A., Robert, G., Locock, L., Sturmey, G., Gager, M., Vougioukalou, S., Ziebland, S., and Fielden, J. (2016) What patients do and their impact on implementation: An ethnographic study of participatory quality improvement projects in English acute hospitals. *Journal of Health Organization and Management* 30(2): 258–278.

Department of Health (1990) *NHS Community and Care Act*. London: The Stationery Office.

Department of Health (1991) *The Patient's Charter*. London: The Stationery Office.

Department of Health (2001a) *Health and Social Care Act* (White Paper). London: The Stationery Office.

Department of Health (2001b) *Involving Patients and Public in Healthcare*. London: The Stationery Office.

Department of Health (2006) *Reward and Recognition: The Principles and Practice of Service User Payment and Reimbursement in Health and Social Care*. 2nd edn. London: The Stationery Office.

Department of Health (2010) *Equity and Excellence: Liberating the NHS*. London: The Stationery Office.

Department of Health (2015) *NHS Constitution*. London: The Stationery Office.

Dr Foster Intelligence (2010) *Intelligent Board 2010 – Patient Experience*. London: Dr Foster Intelligence.

Entwistle, V.A., McCaughan, D., Watt, I.S., Birks, Y., Hall, J., Peat, M., Williams, B, Wright, J. For the Patient Involvement in Patient Safety Group (2010) Speaking up about safety concerns: Multi-setting qualitative study of patients' views and experiences. *Quality and Safety in Health Care* 19: e33.

Evans, D.H., Bacon, R.J., Greer, E., Stagg, A.M., and Turton, P. (2015) 'Calling executives and clinicians to account': User involvement in commissioning cancer services. *Health Expectations* 18(4): 504–515.

Francis, R. (2013) *Report of the Mid Staffordshire NHS Foundation Trust Public Inquiry*. London: The Stationery office.

Martin, G.P. (2008) Representativeness, legitimacy and power in public involvement in health-service management. *Social Science and Medicine* 67: 1757–1765.

NHS Wales (2011) *Learning to Use Patient Stories*. Available from: http://www.1000livespluswales.nhs.uk/ (access on 3 January 2017).

Tollyfield, R. (2014) Facilitating an accelerated experience-based co-design project. *British Journal of Nursing* 23(3): 136–141.

Trier, H., Valderas, J.M., Wensing, M., Martin, H.M., and Egebart, J. (2015) Involving patients in patient safety programmes: A scoping review and consensus procedure by the LINNEAUS collaboration on patient safety in primary care. *European Journal of General Practice* 21(Suppl): 56–61.

Tsianakas, V., Robert, G., Maben, J., Richardson, A., Dale, C., Griffin, M., and Wiseman, T. (2012) Implementing patient-centred cancer care: Using experience-based co-design to improve patient experience in breast and lung cancer services. *Supportive Care in Cancer: Official Journal of the Multinational Association of Supportive Care in Cancer* 20(11): 2639–2647.

5 Ethics and Governance in Healthcare Improvement

Lesley Baillie

Introduction

Ethics is the foundation for quality, and quality improvement must reflect ethical standards, just like clinical care and research (Nelson and Gardent 2008). The word 'ethics' is derived from the Greek word 'ethos' meaning character and is the study of human conduct, principles and behaviour, more specifically their moral behaviour (Baillie and Black 2014). There are various theories of ethics with different frameworks, but in healthcare research, the principles of biomedical ethics (autonomy, non-maleficence, beneficence and justice) (Beauchamp and Childress 2013) are well established and will be examined in relation to quality improvement within this chapter. Nelson et al. (2010) highlighted that these principles underpin the Institute of Medicine's (2001) quality aims for healthcare that are patient-centred, effective, safe, efficient, timely and equitable.

Globally, the principles for conducting research ethically, in particular, that there should be voluntary consent, are well established following the adoption of the World Medical Association's (1964) Declaration of Helsinki. This was the first international standard for biomedical research and led to the setting up of processes for research ethics scrutiny. However, there is less agreement about the application of these processes to quality improvement. Issues include whether quality improvement projects should be reviewed in the same way as research or whether there should be separate, more streamlined systems to prevent delays to improvement activities. This chapter debates these issues, makes suggestions for approaching ethical scrutiny of quality improvement projects and considers their dissemination from an ethical perspective.

Objectives

This chapter's objectives are to:

- Examine the institutional, professional and ethical duty to improve quality in healthcare
- Analyse differences between research and quality improvement and associated influences on ethical considerations and governance
- Discuss potential ethical issues associated with quality improvement, ways of addressing these and processes for ethical approval and governance of quality improvement
- Review the ethical obligation to disseminate quality improvement

The institutional, professional and ethical duty to improve quality in healthcare

Dubler et al. (2007) suggested that institutions are morally obliged to improve quality and to support healthcare professionals to improve quality through creating an enabling environment and infrastructure, monitoring the effectiveness and quality of healthcare practice and making efforts to improve care quality. Similarly, O'Kane (2007) argued that healthcare providers have an ethical responsibility to monitor the care they are delivering and to improve it where it is deficient. In England, the Department of Health's (DH) National Health Service (NHS) Constitution (current version 2015) set out rights and responsibilities for patients and NHS staff with core values that included 'Quality of care'. The core principles include a commitment to service improvement and innovation and to improving services based on feedback. Patients are assured that they can expect

> NHS bodies to monitor, and make efforts to improve continuously, the quality of healthcare they commission or provide. This includes improvements to the safety, effectiveness and experience of services.

(DH 2015, p. 7)

The NHS Constitution also expects healthcare professionals to:

> Play your part in sustainably improving services by working in partnership with patients, the public and communities.

(DH 2015, p. 15)

Healthcare professionals, as individuals, arguably have an ethical responsibility to monitor the care delivered and strive to improve it, thus fulfilling the ethical principle of beneficence (Beauchamp and Childress 2013): actively helping other people. From a nursing perspective, Lang (2007) asserted that ethical concerns for quality healthcare have existed since the time of Florence Nightingale and that nurses have a moral imperative to improve healthcare. Similarly, others have argued that the medical profession has long been committed to improve quality of healthcare (Bellin and Dubler 2001; Wynia and Kurlander 2007). Registered healthcare professionals are accountable to their regulating professional bodies, which sets out requirements of registrants. Box 5.1 includes examples of clauses from three UK professional bodies, presenting the expectation that healthcare professionals will improve quality of care.

However, writing from the United States, Wynia and Kurlander (2007) highlighted that admitting to problems with quality, as a first step in improvement, can be problematic due to concerns such as 'the threat of lawsuits and personal shame'. In England, the NHS Constitution commits to encourage staff to raise any concerns about quality of care though this may not be easy, depending on the context and culture of the organisation concerned. UK healthcare professionals also have a 'duty of candour' and there is a requirement to report adverse events and near misses using established systems (General Medical Council [GMC] and Nursing and Midwifery Council [NMC] 2015). Staff who are leading or managing a team are expected to have systems in place (auditing and benchmarking) to monitor, review and improve the quality of the team's work and as well as individuals having a duty of candour, there is also an organisational duty of candour (GMC and NMC 2015). Dubler et al. (2007) argued that medical professionals are ethically obliged to monitor, reveal and remove medical errors and that each professional is responsible for minimising risk of errors in their own practice. They further

Box 5.1 Healthcare professionals' duty to improve healthcare: Examples from UK professional codes

Nursing and Midwifery Council Code (2015)

8.4 Work with colleagues to evaluate the quality of your work and that of the team (p. 8).

9.2 Gather and reflect on feedback from a variety of sources, using it to improve your practice and performance (p. 8).

25.1 Identify priorities, manage time, staff and resources effectively and deal with risk to make sure that the quality of care or service you deliver is maintained and improved (p. 18).

Health and Care Professions Council: *Standards of Conduct, Performance and Ethics* **(2016)**

3.5 You must ask for feedback and use it to improve your practice.

General Medical Council: *Good Medical Practice* **(2013)**

Contribute to and comply with systems to protect patients.

22. You must take part in systems of quality assurance and quality improvement to promote patient safety. This includes

1   Taking part in regular reviews and audits of your own work and that of your team, responding constructively to the outcomes, taking steps to address any problems and carrying out further training where necessary
2   Regularly reflecting on your standards of practice and the care you provide
3   Reviewing patient feedback where it is available

suggested that whilst not all healthcare professionals can or should conduct quality improvement projects, all should at least support others involved in improving quality. In summary, there is firm agreement that healthcare organisations and professionals have an ethical and professional duty to improve quality in healthcare.

Differentiating between research and quality improvement: The impact on ethical considerations and governance

One key issue that may have an impact on ethical review processes is whether a project is defined as research or quality improvement. Confusion about whether quality improvement is research can cause adverse effects where work should proceed immediately to improve patient safety, whilst also deterring potentially beneficial initiatives because of concerns about burdensome reviews (Davidoff and Batalden 2005; Holm et al. 2007). A project that includes random assignment of standard or alternative treatments or placebos, as in a gold standard, double-blind, randomised controlled trial (RCT), is clearly research and will not resemble a quality improvement project (Bellin and Dubler 2001). However, research that does not use an RCT approach may have some similarity with quality improvement or vice versa, for example, they may use the same data collection methods such as questionnaires, interviews or observation. Other similar attributes between quality improvement and research are that both ask clinically relevant questions and aim for fair selection of participants (Platterborze et al. 2010). Consequently, distinctions between research and quality improvement can become blurred (Lynn 2004; O'Kane 2007; Holm et al. 2007).

The Hastings Center in the United States convened leaders and scholars to address ethical requirements for quality improvement and their relationship to regulations protecting human research participants (Lynn et al. 2007). The group defined quality improvement as 'systematic, data-guided activities designed to bring about immediate improvements in healthcare delivery in particular settings' (p. 667) and concluded that quality improvement is an intrinsic part of normal healthcare operations, whilst research is not an obligation and so a person's decision to participate in research must be voluntary and fully informed to prevent exploitation. Platterborze et al. (2010) identified differences as follows:

- **Quality improvement:** Incorporates ongoing modification of the project, involves usual care, evaluates procedures of no more than minimum risk and involves people working in a local context
- **Research:** Tests knowledge beyond what is known (e.g., trying out a new intervention), uses randomisation of patients, includes a deliberate delay in results being fed back to prevent potential bias in interpretation and is often externally funded

In practice however, projects may not be as clear cut as this, for example, quality improvement might be funded and could occur at more than local level, research does not always involve randomisation and so on. The World Health Organisation (WHO) (2013) identified that activities that do not meet the criteria for research may still pose more than minimal risk, which may be context-specific and so it is important to understand the organisational culture, for example will there be retribution if errors are exposed? Can confidentiality be assured? The WHO (2013) recommended independent ethical oversight wherever more than minimum risk is identified, pointing out that no matter how the activity is labelled, what is important is that people are not subjected to risk as risks can generally be anticipated and strategies planned to deal with them.

In England, the Health Research Authority (HRA) is a national body responsible for governance of research in the NHS. The organisation defines research and provides a decision tool to assist project leads in deciding whether their project is research, from an NHS research ethics perspective (see http://www.hra.nhs.uk/research-community/before-you-apply /determine-whether-your-study-is-research/) or whether it is audit, surveillance, public health or service evaluation, which the HRA states may include service improvement or quality improvement. If the project does not meet the criteria for research (randomisation, use of treatment/care different from usual standard, intention to derive generalisable new knowledge) then it will not require an NHS research ethics committee review although other local governance processes may be needed within the NHS (Health Research Authority 2016). Thus the decision about whether a project constitutes research or quality improvement affects whether the project undergoes a research ethics committee review or other governance process. Internationally, there have been assertions that project leads may deliberately put across projects as quality improvement, rather than research, in order to avoid the burden of research ethical review, which is considered time-consuming and onerous (Horsfall and Cleary 2002; Lynn 2004; Grady 2007; Eccles et al. 2011). Such a strategy highlights dissatisfaction with existing research ethics review processes but the consequent lack of ethical scrutiny is of concern.

Lynn et al. (2007) suggested that the confusion about whether a quality improvement project comes under research governance regulations relates mainly to how the phrase 'designed to develop or contribute to generalisable knowledge' is interpreted. The Hastings Center project group concluded that generalisability should be defined in a narrow way, meaning that most quality improvement projects would not qualify as research (Lynn et al. 2007). However, if a quality improvement activity is designed both to improve local care and to produce broadly generalisable knowledge, it is both quality improvement and research (Lynn et al. 2007). Writing from a U.S. perspective, Fiscella et al. (2015) reported that Institutional Review Boards (IRBs) define research on the basis of rigorous methods and generalisability of the knowledge gained. However, they pointed out that methods used should be rigorous regardless of whether activities are defined as quality improvement or research. The nature of generalisability is not clear-cut as healthcare quality improvement studies often produce results that can be generalisable or are of interest to others even if that is not the primary purpose (Byers and Aragon 2003; Dubler et al. 2007). As an example, the WHO's Surgical Checklist, which was a quality improvement initiative to eliminate errors associated with surgery, is used internationally (Haynes et al. 2011); see Box 3.1 in Chapter 3, for more details. Furthermore, Fiscella et al. (2015) questioned the generalisability of traditional RCTs, which often have highly selective samples, exclude patients with any comorbidities and are conducted in specialist settings. In contrast, quality improvement involves 'real-world settings' with more inclusive samples, and most findings could be generalisable beyond the participants, healthcare delivery systems and practice settings involved (Fiscella et al. 2015). Whether quality improvement work is generalisable may depend on the specific context and unique features of the organisation in which it takes place (Fiscella et al. 2015). Thus generalisability may be difficult to ascertain at the start of a project but even within the same healthcare system, there may be different sites and varied settings where the findings from quality improvement activities could be applied.

In summary, whilst there have been many attempts to differentiate between research and quality improvement, there are clearly blurred areas and consequently practitioners can feel unclear about whether their quality improvement project needs submission to a research ethics review (Tapp et al. 2009). For quality improvement, ethics review processes need to be able to deal with projects that have a more flexible design than traditional research and review projects in a timely way that does not pose a barrier to quality improvement. Davidoff and Batalden (2005) emphasised that what matters is whether staff engaged in improvement have taken the appropriate steps to protect people who participate, rather than whether they are doing research.

Ethical issues associated with quality improvement

Like all aspects of healthcare practice and management, improvement activities must be sensitive to the rights and interests of patients and be conducted in an ethically responsible manner (Jennings et al. 2007). The WHO (2013) identified that quality improvement and research share many similar features (e.g., use of patient data) and so therefore raise similar ethical concerns. In terms of the Helsinki principles, Doyal (2004) argued that whilst the risks of quality improvement may be less than those arising in some conventional healthcare research, there are still risks, for example confidentiality of patients or staff may be breached or the wording of questionnaires could be distressing. Other potential ethical issues arise because improvement activities may inadvertently cause harm, waste scarce resources or affect some patients unfairly (Lynn et al. 2007); these are examples of how the principles of bioethics can be contravened in quality improvement (e.g., non-maleficence, justice). In the United States, Taylor et al. (2010) surveyed quality improvement practitioners involved in the Institute of Health Improvement's 100,000 lives campaign and found that they strongly agreed that ensuring minimum risk and

Table 5.1 Principles of bioethics, with quality improvement (QI) examples

Principle	Definition	Quality improvement example
Autonomy	Self-government or self-determination	Participant can choose whether to take part in quality improvement based on accurate information
Non-maleficence	We must cause no harm to others: 'one ought not to inflict evil or harm' (p. 152)	Participant is assured that their confidentiality will be maintained thus not causing embarrassment
Beneficence	Actively taking positive steps to help others and contribute to their welfare	Rigorous conduct of the quality improvement activity, leads to benefits and learning
Justice	What is right and fair	Patients and staff have an equitable opportunity to take part in quality improvement and are not unfairly excluded

Source: Adapted from Beauchamp, T.L. and Childress, F., *Principles of Biomedical Ethics*, 7th edn., Oxford University Press, Oxford, 2013.

confidentiality were relevant considerations in quality improvement. Most also agreed that assessing existing practices, a scientifically sound design, transparency and identifying and minimising potential conflicts, were important ethical concerns.

Beauchamp and Childress's (2013) principles of bioethics are summarised in Table 5.1 and are next discussed in relation to quality improvement.

Autonomy

Autonomy is a core ethical principle and in bioethics means self-government or self-determination, as it comes from the Greek words 'autos' meaning self and 'nomos' meaning law, governance or rule. Beauchamp and Childress (2013) define autonomy as:

> self-rule that is free from both controlling interference by others and limitations that prevent meaningful choice, such as inadequate understanding. The autonomous individual acts freely in accordance with a self-chosen plan. (p. 101)

Beauchamp and Childress (2013, p. 104) presented three conditions for autonomous choice: intentionality (acting according to a plan), understanding (of the choice to be made) and non-control (the choice being made free from control by external or internal influences).

Autonomy as a core ethical principle underpins the current emphasis on informed consent: making the choice about engaging in treatment or care (Holm et al. 2007). Informed consent is intended to protect participants from exposure to additional risks posed by research that they have not agreed to and that goes beyond the usual standard of clinical care, whilst respecting their autonomy and preferences (Miller and Emmanuel 2008). There are rigorous processes for informed consent in research, including clear information that is communicated in an accessible way and sufficient time to decide whether to take part. Particular care must be followed with vulnerable populations (e.g., children, people with learning disabilities and people with impaired mental capacity). However, there is a risk that because of the challenges present in gaining informed consent, more vulnerable populations may be given less opportunity to take part in research, which has further ethical connotations: a risk of removing autonomy (lack of choice to decide whether to participate) as well as countering the principle of justice. Newhouse et al. (2006) clarified that written consent is required for research as it does not usually directly benefit the participants but can be burdensome and pose risks to them.

There has been considerable debate about how the principle of autonomy and informed consent applies to involvement of patients and staff in quality improvement activities (Fiscella et al. 2015). For example, Bellin and Dubler (2001) argued that quality improvement is ethically intrinsic to care provision and so the notion of informed consent is irrelevant. A further argument is that patients have a responsibility to take part as the delivery of reliably high-quality healthcare depends on all patients' participation (Lynn et al. 2007). However, Lynn et al. (2007) clarified that this responsibility is subject to standards of reasonableness: that patients have access to general information about improvement activities and are kept safe from harm and from infringements of their rights. For example, both patients and staff should be assured of confidentiality and have the opportunity to choose whether to participate in an improvement activity that presents more than minimal risk. Risks may pertain to clinical, psychological, social or economic aspects and 'minimal risk' is considered to be no more than risk incurred in routine daily life or routine healthcare examination or for staff, risk that is encountered in routine daily practice (WHO 2013). Lynn et al. (2007) suggested that individual informed consent should be obtained for improvement activities that entail more than minimal risk, for example, additional physical or psychological harm, burden related to the change itself or to surveys or medical procedures required for monitoring.

In Tapp et al.'s (2009) study, European general practitioners (GPs) questioned whether patients had any choice about participating in quality improvement but they were also concerned that gaining consent from individuals for every quality improvement project was too time consuming and difficult. Dubler et al. (2007) presented a number of arguments against obtaining individual informed consent in quality improvement activities: patients' non-participation could lead to wasted healthcare resources as improvements cannot be made; patients may experience immediate benefit from quality improvement (unlike in research); improvement involves patients receiving ongoing care (they are not randomised to different treatments); risks are usually minimal, and a fully informed consent process would delay or prevent improvement activity, with potentially adverse effects on quality.

One suggestion is for universal consent: informing all new patients about improvement activities within the institution (Dubler et al. 2007; Holm et al. 2007; Fiscella et al. 2015). Indeed, Lynn et al. (2007) argued that consent to receive care should include consent to participate in routine, minimal-risk quality improvement activities. An example could include the auditing of patient records for antibiotic prescribing so that practices can be improved. Fiscella et al. (2015) suggested that there could be opt-out opportunities for patients in quality improvement activities; this would entail patients being informed that, for example, all records are being examined for quality purposes and that if they do not wish their records to be used for this purpose they can decline. However, further issues then arise such as ensuring all patients, regardless of their health condition, have the information needed to decide to opt-out; potentially people without the mental capacity to make such a decision would be excluded.

A form of universal consent seems to have been adopted by the NHS Constitution in England (DH 2015), which pledges to:

> anonymise the information collected during the course of your treatment and use it to support research and improve care for others. (p. 8)

This approach reflects the view that individual informed consent is not required for improvement activities that involve patient data as long as these data are adequately protected to maintain individual privacy (Dubler et al. 2007). Whilst this stance provides a lack of choice for individuals about the use of their data for research and quality improvement, it could be argued on the grounds of other ethical principles that if data are anonymised, there can be no harm (non-maleficence), and there is potential to improve care (beneficence). However, in Tapp et al.'s (2009) study, GPs identified concerns about use of data for quality improvement; issues included use of data collected for one purpose being used in a different way without consent. Some GPs raised the concern that technological advances enabled the easy sharing of data across settings but that, 'Partly we do it because we can. It doesn't mean we should'. The GPs agreed that there should be more transparency about how GPs use data with suggestions for a generalised gaining of consent. O'Kane (2007) argued that informed consent is not just about protecting individuals from risks; it provides the right to self-determination so individuals can choose what shall or shall not happen to them. For example, where interviews or questionnaires are used as part of data collection in quality improvement, patients should be informed as to how the information will be used and given the opportunity to decline to take part.

Non-maleficence

The Hippocratic requirement for the medical profession is 'primum non nocere', meaning, 'Above all [or first] do no harm' and other health professionals' codes of ethics set out similar expectations. This reflects the principle of non-maleficence meaning that we must cause no harm to others: 'one ought not to inflict evil or harm' (Beauchamp and Childress 2013, p. 152). Holm et al. (2007) asserted that whilst quality improvement activities usually carry the same level of risk as delivering standard care there can be some specific risks, particularly where improvement work is of poor quality and under-resourced. O'Kane (2007) goes further and identified that patients could be harmed, albeit not deliberately, if quality improvement projects are badly planned and managed and involve 'poorly conceived quality interventions by inadequately supervised practitioners' (O'Kane 2007, p. 93). Davidoff (2007) highlighted various factors that affect the potential for harm from quality improvement: how much the improved practice differs from established evidence and current standards; the number of people who might be affected by the change; the effect size and efficacy of the intervention proposed; and what is known or can be predicted, about any risks, their potential for harm, and hence the need for protection.

O'Kane (2007) argued that alongside an ethical responsibility to undertake improvement, practitioners must manage and conduct improvement effectively, thus preventing harm. Factors increasing risk of harm are instances where governance and accountability are unclear (highlighting the need for scrutiny) and the short duration of projects (linked to funding) with a lack of structures to sustain improvement. Like research, any quality improvement project involves use of resources and potential burden and risk (however small) to participants – service users and staff – which cannot be justified if the findings are invalid due to a design that lacks rigour (Fiscella et al. 2015). Strategies to reduce risk include learning from prior implementation of similar changes in other settings (thus highlighting an ethical duty to publish improvement projects), starting small-scale, closely monitoring effects of changes and revising innovations to limit adverse effects (Lynn 2004). Finally, we should also recognise that:

while quality improvement might pose an undue risk, patients receiving care in a setting that accepts mediocre results poses risks to their well-being that are real and substantial and likely of much greater magnitude.

(O'Kane 2007, p. 98)

In essence, not conducting and supporting activities to improve healthcare certainly has potential to cause harm. Nevertheless, we must ensure that quality improvement activities are conducted to the highest standard possible, thus supporting the ethical principle of beneficence.

Beneficence

Whilst non-maleficence requires that we should do no harm, beneficence requires us to actively take positive steps to help others and contribute to their welfare (Beauchamp and Childress 2013). Holm et al. (2007) identified that quality improvement in general, as part of clinical practice, aims to improve patient care and safety by maximising patient benefit (beneficence) whilst minimising patient harm and risk (non-maleficence). There are many examples of improvement activities that have led to tangible benefits for patients, for example, a quality improvement project significantly reduced pressure ulcer risk in a paediatric intensive care unit (Visscher et al. 2013). Holm et al. (2007) maintained that benefits are more likely to be achieved where the practitioner shows professional integrity and conducts honest collection and reporting of data, including reasonable judgments about the project's value for the care setting and the organisation as a whole, use of appropriate metrics to measure improvement, adequate data collection for what is being examined, sufficient resources to conduct and complete the project and use of informed consent as necessary, with appropriate ethical scrutiny. Thus conducting quality improvement activities to a high standard will be more likely to have positive outcomes and improvements that benefit healthcare. Furthermore, quality improvement activities must be disseminated effectively so that they can benefit others too (see The ethical obligation to disseminate healthcare improvement and Chapter 9).

Justice

In alignment with the meaning of justice more widely, justice in the healthcare context is about what is right and fair. The principle is closely linked to equality and in relation to quality improvement, concerns fair opportunity to participate in and to benefit from quality improvement activities. Holm et al. (2007) argued that for quality improvement activities, the principle of justice should guide not only the selection and inclusion process related to participants whose activities or data will be observed or collected (i.e., patients, family members, employees) but also project leaders and team members who need access to organisational resources (e.g., money, personnel) to initiate and complete their projects. The selection of quality improvement projects to pursue must also adhere to the principle of justice. In Tapp et al.'s (2009) study, GPs felt it important that there was transparency about how projects were prioritised, but they identified potential influences on project choices, including government policy, society, drug companies or insurance companies. In addition, they highlighted that there may be financial incentives for GPs to conduct quality improvement, rather than being motivated to improve care, with less time spent on individual patients as a result. They considered that some projects might be prioritised as they are easier to conduct than others that may be more necessary and lead to greater benefit (beneficence).

Identifying and addressing ethical issues in quality improvement

Table 5.2 sets out ethical requirements for protecting participants in quality improvement activities, adapted from Lynn et al. (2007), who reported on the work by the United States' Hastings Center. The requirements are linked to the bioethical principles (Beauchamp and Childress 2013).

Wade (2007) argued for the need to ensure that the collection and analysis of data for quality improvement is conducted ethically, with the key question being what is the goal of the quality improvement activity and how will risks and benefits be balanced? He presented a list of questions to be asked with any improvement project (see Box 5.2). He argued that organisations and the people involved are responsible for ethical collection and analysis of patient data but that processes should not lead to barriers. For any practitioner planning a quality improvement project, these questions pose a useful framework for ethical considerations. However, practitioners must also consider independent review of their proposed project and ethical scrutiny.

Ethical scrutiny and governance of quality improvement activities

O'Kane (2007) argued that if there is an ethical responsibility to undertake quality improvement, there is also a responsibility to manage and conduct it effectively and well and ensure that the institution has a rigorous and strategic agenda to improve the quality of its care. She suggested that quality improvement should be overseen by a responsible structure, accountable to senior management and institutional governance, in order to protect patients from ad hoc or poorly conceived quality improvement projects. However, Taylor et al. (2010) identified that whilst most quality improvement activities had some ethical scrutiny, this was often not independent of those conducting the improvement, implying that an institutional approach and independent review were lacking. This situation contrasts sharply with the well-established processes for formal ethical scrutiny and approval of research by an ethics committee prior to the research starting, resulting from the Declaration of Helsinki (Eccles et al. 2011). Lynn (2004) identified that these research ethical scrutiny processes were developed to 'guard against people being tricked into taking risks for the benefit of "science", "researchers" or generally "other people" in the future' (p. 69).

For any practitioner planning to undertake quality improvement activities and projects, navigating ethical approvals is an important consideration, but processes for ethical scrutiny are often not clear cut. One reason is that, as discussed earlier, the differentiation between what is research and what is quality improvement is contentious. In addition, processes for reviewing quality improvement as distinct from research are not well established in many areas. The result is that quality improvement projects may be reviewed using the same process as for research and this may be disproportionate, leading to delays in starting improvement activity (Lynn 2004). The need for ethical scrutiny of quality improvement to be proportionate is therefore highlighted, with comments that patients need more protection in healthcare systems that are not actively engaged in quality improvement than in systems that are (Davidoff and Batalden 2005). Similarly, Lynn et al. (2007) asserted that the overall approach to ethical scrutiny of quality improvement should acknowledge that the risks to participants are regularly less than the risks from allowing quality and safety deficits to persist or introducing changes without monitoring their effects.

In contrast, if the project is considered not to be research and there is no alternative review facility for quality improvement, it may receive no independent review at all, even though there are at least minimal risks in any quality improvement project. Flaming et al. (2009)

Table 5.2 Ethical requirements for protecting participants in quality improvement in healthcare

Requirement	Bioethical principle	Explanation
Social or scientific value	Non-maleficence Beneficence	The gains from the quality improvement activity should justify resources used and risks imposed on participants.
Scientific validity	Beneficence	A quality improvement activity should be methodologically sound (i.e., appropriately structured to achieve its goals).
Fair participant selection	Justice	Selection of participants should achieve a fair distribution of burdens and benefits of quality improvement.
Favourable risk–benefit ratio	Non-maleficence Beneficence	A quality improvement activity should be designed to limit risks whilst maximising potential benefits and to ensure that risks to individual participants are balanced by expected benefits to the participant and society.
Respect for participants	Non-maleficence	A quality improvement activity should be designed to protect the privacy of participants and confidentiality of their personal information.
	Beneficence	Participants should receive information about findings from quality improvement activities that are clinically relevant to their own care.
	Autonomy	All patients and staff in a care setting should receive basic information about quality improvement activities.
		The results from quality improvement should be shared with others in the healthcare system but participant confidentiality must be protected by putting results into non-identifiable form or obtaining specific consent to sharing.
Informed consent	Autonomy Non-maleficence	Consent to inclusion in minimal-risk quality improvement activities is part of the patient's consent to treatment.
		Workers (employees or non-employee professionals who provide care in an organisation) should participate in minimal-risk quality improvement activities as part of their job responsibilities.
		Patients and workers should be asked for informed consent to be included in a specific quality improvement activity if it imposes more than minimal risk: the risk to patients should be measured relative to the risk associated with receiving standard care whilst the risk to workers should be measured relative to the risk associated with the usual work situation.
Independent review	Non-maleficence Beneficence	Accountability for the ethical conduct of quality improvement should be integrated into practices that ensure accountability for clinical care. Each quality improvement activity should receive the kind of ethical review and supervision that is appropriate to its level of potential risk and project worth.

Source: Adapted from Lynn, J. et al., *Ann Intern Med.*, 146, 666–673, 2007.

provided an example of a quality improvement project in Canada, illustrating the project leader's awareness of the associated ethical issues, which appear to be more than minimal, and yet there was no facility for an ethical review as the project was not research (see Box 5.3).

Box 5.2 Questions to consider in relation to any systematic data collection in healthcare

Design

Will the design answer the question being asked?

Process

- How much will each participant be informed about the study?
- Will each participant be able to choose whether or not to participate?
- Will the method of recruiting participants be fair?

Cost

- What organisational resources will this project use?
- What extra burden will be imposed on the participant(s)?
- What additional risks will the participant(s) face?

Benefits

- What benefit might accrue to the participant(s)?
- What benefit might accrue to society?

Source: Wade, D., *Br Med J.*, 334, 1330–1331, 2007.

Box 5.3 A quality improvement project and ethical issues

The quality improvement project involved moving a harm reduction programme for intravenous users out of an inner city area, with a plan to collect data through interviews with two groups of people: those who had used the service but whose access had now changed, and those people living near the new site. The users of the service included sex workers, people with addictions, mental health conditions or impaired cognitive function; many were vulnerable and marginalised. Following local screening, the project was identified as quality improvement rather than research and the leaders were advised that it could not be reviewed by the research ethics committee. There was no alternative ethics committee available. Yet, the project leader identified a number of ethical issues: the participants were vulnerable and marginalised and could feel coercion to take part, the interview topics were likely to be sensitive and could cause upset (e.g., sexual orientation, illegal substances), a breach of confidentiality could affect employment or reputation and capacity to consent could be impaired in some individuals.

Source: Adapted from Flaming, D. et al., *Healthc Q.*, 12, 52–57, 2009.

Ethical scrutiny processes for quality improvement

Wise (2007) referred to the imperfect match between quality improvement activities and the existing institutional research ethics boards as a 'forced marriage'. Concerns about research ethics committees as a way of reviewing quality improvement include their inability to deal with rapid changes, small samples and limited documentation and the requirement for rigid research protocols (Lynn 2004). There is concern that the disproportionately large resources needed to prepare a research ethics submission may inhibit project developments (Lynn et al. 2007). Jennings et al. (2007) questioned whether, conceptually and practically, research ethics committees are the most effective and reasonable way to ensure that quality improvement is carried out ethically and that they may inadvertently undermine the protection of patient interests. Others have argued that research ethics committees are already overstretched and adding quality improvement projects to their work would be burdensome and decrease effectiveness (Doyal 2004; Flaming et al. 2009). However, one journal's editors has questioned how professionals make their decisions about seeking ethics reviews, arguing that there must be a local standard that has been applied as 'unilateral judgments by authors not to seek ethics review are potentially self-serving' (*BMJ Quality and Safety* 2014).

Overall, there is much agreement that research ethics processes may not serve quality improvement well. There is strong support, however, for independent reviews of quality improvement projects, in order to protect the rights of those who receive and deliver healthcare, but with flexible, proportionate and quick review systems that do not pose barriers to design and implementation (Doyal 2004; Dubler et al. 2007; Grady 2007; Bottrell 2007; Holm et al. 2007; Flaming et al. 2009). Separate ethics review processes for quality improvement may therefore be preferable (Bellin and Dubler 2001; Dubler et al. 2007; Flaming et al. 2009). Bottrell (2007) suggested 'Quality-Improvement Review Committees' with members who are knowledgeable about quality improvement techniques and associated ethical standards and access to individuals with specific knowledge of the practice area that will undergo improvement. Fiscella et al. (2015) made suggestions for a review process for quality improvement, arguing that an initial rapid review would minimise the risk of projects being considered 'exempt' from full review without there being auditable documentation of minimal, independent review (see Box 5.4). Fiscella et al. (2015) argued that such a system would balance the

---

Box 5.4 Proposal for ethical review committees for quality improvement

- A short application (succinct one page document that summarises key ethical considerations), quicker turn-around times and a two-stage review process
- An initial review within a few days with either approval of the project or referral for further committee review
- Independent review to include perspectives from people with appropriate expertise in the methods, including, clinicians, service users and people with ethical expertise
- Review to consider whether methods are sufficiently rigorous to meet the project's goals and help to ensure appropriate use of resources, as well as protection of people's privacy and safety

Source: Adapted from Fiscella, K. et al., *BMC Med Ethics*, 16, 63, 2015.

protection of participants' rights with the ethical requirement to improve care as rapidly as possible by building a healthcare system that continuously learns from its data.

Wise (2008) reported on the setting up of an ethics scrutiny process based on the work of the Hastings Center (Lynn et al. 2007; Jennings et al. 2007) and asserted that the process enriched their organisation's quality improvement activities without curtailing them. Flaming et al. (2009) reported that the Alberta Research Ethics Community Consensus Initiative (ARECCI) network have developed ethics guidelines for quality improvement projects with six considerations, based on the Hastings Center work. Table 5.3 presents six questions to ask with the rationale; the website (see http://www.aihealthsolutions.ca/arecci/guidelines/) sets these out as an online tool with points to consider for each question and screening of level of risk based on responses. Flaming et al. (2009) suggested that anyone conducting quality improvement should use the guidelines from the start of planning the project. The tool has been pilot tested as a decision support guide.

Table 5.3 ARECCI's six ethical considerations in planning a QI project

Question	Rationale
How will the knowledge gained from this project be useful?	A QI project can only be justified if the results are immediately useful or will be in the near future in a specific context. Asking for participation in an unnecessary project wastes limited time and resources whilst exposing participants to unnecessary risks.
How will the described method or approach generate the desired knowledge?	Consider whether any methods will lead to identification of participants and how it will be decided that enough data is collected (as data must be on a 'need-to-know' basis). A sound method is more likely to lead to reliable information. Badly designed projects waste limited time and resources.
How will you ensure that the participant (or data) selection process is fair and appropriate?	Most appropriate participants are key stakeholders. Must avoid overburdening particular groups. Need to consider safeguarding of people's privacy and human rights.
What have you done to identify and minimise risks as well as maximise benefits? Are the remaining risks justified?	Few projects are completely risk free from the perspectives of individuals or the organisation. Examples include risk of breaching confidentiality, a person feeling coerced to take part, or the results leading to adverse consequences for a participant or the organisation. Potential risks must be clearly identified, minimised (reduce or prevent likelihood of occurrence) or mitigated (ease or make less severe if occurs). The risks must be balanced with potential benefits.
How are the rights of individuals, communities and populations respected in this project?	Impact on privacy and confidentiality: storage of data, how long data is collected, who will access the data and whether participants will be informed of the results.
Is informed consent needed in this project?	Asking for consent in some projects could be burdensome. Broad consent for individuals entering a service may be more appropriate. Examples of projects needing consent are those involving a power relationship between the person collecting the data and the participant, those in which there might be a conflict of interest or where more than minimal risk has been identified.

Source: Adapted from Flaming, D. et al., *Healthc Q.*, 12, 53–54, 2009.

Planning ethical scrutiny for your quality improvement project

Whilst in many instances, quality improvement activities may have minimal associated risk, the important factor is that you carefully consider what the risks are and how these can be addressed. You may find it useful to use the HRA's decision tree (referred to earlier) to determine if your project would be considered 'research' and will require a research ethics application process, in addition to any other organisational and university requirements.

You may find that the local processes for review of quality improvement are not conducive to the rapid, informed and proportionate review that would be ideal. You may be expected to submit your project through a research ethics review process or be informed that, as the project is quality improvement, it does not need formal review. You must follow the ethical governance requirements of your organisation and (if applicable) the university where you are studying. You may also be in a position to suggest alternative and more appropriate review processes, based on this chapter's information. We suggest that you use ARECCI's six ethical considerations for quality improvement (see Table 5.3) to review the project during planning. In summary, we suggest the following:

If your project is being conducted as part of a university course

1 Check your healthcare organisation's ethics and governance guidance. They may require that your project is reviewed by an organisational department or committee prior to university ethical approval. Your university may then only require a copy of the organisational approval, rather than conducting another review. Alternatively, as your project is quality improvement, your organisation may not require an ethical review. They may ask you to register your project as a quality improvement project in the organisation or they may not have any requirements of you.

2 Check the university's requirements. It is likely that you must complete a university ethics application and your project will be reviewed by a university committee, which may handle both research and quality improvement and other practice-based projects. Your university will usually require written evidence that your organisation supports the project and that you have permission to proceed. They may also require a written statement confirming that your healthcare organisation does not require the project to undergo their institutional research ethics review, if that is what they advised.

If your project is not being conducted as part of a university course

1 Check your healthcare organisation's ethics and governance requirements. They may require that your project is reviewed by an organisational department or committee. However, as your project is quality improvement, your organisation may not require an ethical review. They may require you to register your quality improvement project in the organisation or they not have any requirements of you.

2 If your organisation does not offer any ethical review for quality improvement, there may be another forum where your project plan can be reviewed. Otherwise, ask for an independent review by an appropriate colleague who is not involved in the project and record that this has taken place. They could use ARECCI's six ethical considerations (Table 5.3) as the basis for their review.

Box 5.5 Consequences of not publishing quality improvement

- Prevents assessment of potential for repeatability of the quality improvement activities and prevents further learning
- Prevents critical public debate (e.g., though peer review, editorial input, readers' letters and debates, and hence accountability)
- Reduces the incentive and opportunity to clarify thinking, verify observations and justify inferences, which occur while writing up results for publication
- Slows the dissemination of known effective innovations and wastes the time, effort and money that others spend independently rediscovering those same innovations – and making the same mistakes
- Slows the development of improvement science, since dissemination of information about one innovation sparks others

Source: Adapted from Davidoff, F. and Batalden, P., *Qual Saf Health Care*, 14, 319–325, 2005.

The ethical obligation to disseminate healthcare improvement

Chapter 9 considers in detail, the different options for ensuring that the outcomes and learning from quality improvement are disseminated effectively. Here, we consider the ethical obligation to disseminate quality improvement work, with a particular focus on publication, which can ensure that it is widely available. The reasons for not publishing quality improvement work may include competing service responsibilities and lack of academic rewards for improvement, staff, editors' and peer reviewers' unfamiliarity with improvement goals and methods, and lack of publication guidelines that are appropriate for rigorous, scholarly improvement work (Davidoff and Batalden 2005). Nevertheless, Davidoff and Batalden (2005) highlighted that quality improvement uses public resources and exposes participants to inconvenience, cost and risk and therefore failure to share the results of improvement work publicly, in return for those contributions, should be challenged on ethical grounds. Furthermore, they identify a range of adverse effects of not publishing improvement work (see Box 5.5). Whilst generalisation may not be a goal of quality improvement, project findings could be informative to other organisations with similar patient populations (Dubler et al. 2007). Holm et al. (2007) too argued that lack of publication results in a lack of scrutiny, and improvements in quality improvement methodologies are slowed because ideas are not shared. Conversely, quality improvement projects that are widely disseminated could have skewed results and ethical problems, highlighting that critical review by readers, as well as during the peer review publication process, is essential. In addition, readers should be aware that in some improvement initiatives, there may have been an upward secular trend with improvement that is already happening, outside the improvement intervention.

Conclusion

Healthcare professionals have a professional and ethical duty to provide high-quality care based on best evidence and to improve care delivery using rigorous approaches. Improving quality involves changing practice so there will always be some risk that needs to be weighed up against the risk of not taking action to improve quality. The bioethical principles of autonomy, non-maleficence, beneficence and justice, which are commonly used in ethical review of research are also applicable to quality improvement. During the planning of improvement activities, associated ethical implications must be identified and addressed and an independent ethical review should be conducted, which may also enhance the project design. However, institutional processes for reviewing quality improvement may be lacking, and there can be confusion about whether a project is considered research or quality improvement. The application of research ethics review processes may delay improvement activity, but there may be no alternative ethics review process available for quality improvement projects. However, the individual leading a quality improvement activity has an ethical duty to ensure that ethical review has been conducted, and this chapter suggested frameworks to support independent ethical review. Finally, there is an ethical duty to disseminate quality improvement to enable learning and wider application where appropriate.

References

Baillie, L. and Black, S. (2014) *Professional Values in Nursing*. London: Taylor & Francis.

Beauchamp, T.L. and Childress, F. (2013) *Principles of Biomedical Ethics*, 7th edn. Oxford: Oxford University Press.

Bellin, E. and Dubler, N.N. (2001) The quality improvement–research divide and the need for external oversight. *American Journal of Public Health* 91(9): 1512–1517.

BMJ Quality and Safety (2014) Policy on ethics review for quality improvement projects. Available from: http://qualitysafety.bmj.com

Bottrell, M.M. (2007) Accountability for the conduct of quality-improvement projects1. In: Jennings, B., Baily, M.A., Bottrell, M., Lynn, J., editors. *Quality Health Care Quality Improvement: Ethical and Regulatory Issues*. New York, NY: The Hastings Center, pp. 129–144.

Byers, J.F. and Aragon, E.D. (2003) What quality improvement professionals need to know about IRBs. *Journal for Healthcare Quality* 25(4): 4–9.

Davidoff, F. (2007) Publication and the ethics of quality improvement. In: Jennings, B., Baily, M.A., Bottrell, M., Lynn, J., editors. *Health Care Quality Improvement: Ethical and Regulatory Issues*. New York, NY: The Hastings Center, pp. 101–106.

Davidoff, F. and Batalden, P. (2005) Toward stronger evidence on quality improvement. Draft publication guidelines: The beginning of a consensus project. *Quality and Safety in Health Care* 14(5): 319–325.

Department of Health (2015) *The NHS Constitution for England*. England: Department of Health. Available from: https://www.gov.uk/government/publications/the-nhs-constitution-for-england (accessed on 1 April 2016).

Doyal, L. (2004) Preserving moral quality in research, audit, and quality improvement. *Quality and Safety in Health Care* 13(1): 11–12.

Dubler, N., Blustein, J., Bhalla, R., and Bernard, D. (2007) Informed participation: An alternative ethical process for including patients in quality-improvement projects. In: Jennings, B., Baily, M.A., Bottrell, M., Lynn, J., editors. *Quality Health Care Quality Improvement: Ethical and Regulatory Issues*. New York, NY: The Hastings Center, pp. 69–87.

Eccles, M.P., Weijer, C., and Mittman, B. (2011) Requirements for ethics committee review for studies submitted to implementation. *Implementation Science* 6: 32.

Fiscella, K., Tobin, J.N., Carroll, J.K., He, H., and Ogedegbe, G. (2015) Ethical oversight in quality improvement and quality improvement research: New approaches to promote a learning health care system. *BMC Medical Ethics* 16(1): 63.

Flaming, D., Barratt-Smith, L., and Brown, N. (2009) Ethics? But its only quality improvement. *Healthcare Quarterly* 12(2): 52–57.

General Medical Council (2013) *Good Medical Practice*. Available from: http://www.gmc-uk.org/guidance/good_medical_practice/systems_protect.asp (accessed on 1 April 2016).

General Medical Council and Nursing and Midwifery Council (2015) *Openness and Honesty When Things Go Wrong: The Professional Duty of Candour*. Available from: http://www.gmc-uk.org/DoC _ guidance_englsih.pdf_61618688.pdf (accessed on 22 June 2016).

Grady, C. (2007) Quality improvement and ethical oversight. *Annals of Internal Medicine* 146(9): 680–681.

Haynes, A.B., Weiser, T.G., Berry, W.R., Lipsitz, S.R., Breizat, A.H., Dellinger E.P., et al. (2011) Changes in safety attitude and relationship to decreased postoperative morbidity and mortality following implementation of a checklist-based surgical safety intervention. *BMJ Quality and Safety* 20(1); 102–107.

Health and Care Professions Council (2016) *Standards of Conduct, Performance and Ethics*. Available from: http://www.hpc-uk.org/aboutregistration/standards/standardsofconductperformanceandethics/ (accessed on 1 April 2016).

Health Research Authority (2016) *Defining Research*. Available from: http://www.hra.nhs.uk/documents/2016/06/defining-research.pdf (accessed on 17 August 2016).

Holm, M.J., Selvan, M., Smith, M.L., Markman, M., Theriault, R., Rodriguez, M.A., and Martin, S. (2007) Quality improvement or research: Defining and supervising QI at the University of Texas M. D. Anderson cancer center. In: Jennings, B, Baily, M.A., Bottrell, M., Lynn, J., editors. *Quality Health Care Quality Improvement: Ethical and Regulatory Issues*. New York, NY: The Hastings Center, pp. 145–168.

Horsfall, J. and Cleary, M. (2002) Mental health quality improvement: What about ethics? *International Journal of Mental Health Nursing* 11(1): 40–46.

Institute of Medicine. (2001) *Committee on Quality of Healthcare in America. Crossing the Quality Chasm: A New Health System for the 21st Century*. Washington, DC: National Academy Press.

Jennings, B., Baily, M.A., Bottrell, M., and Lynn, J. (2007) Introduction. In: Jennings B., Baily M.A., Bottrell M., Lynn J., editors. *Quality Health Care Quality Improvement: Ethical and Regulatory Issues*. New York, NY: The Hastings Center, pp. 29–53.

Lang, N.M. (2007) Health care quality improvement: A nursing perspective. In: Jennings B., Baily M.A., Bottrell M., Lynn J., editors. *Quality Health Care Quality Improvement: Ethical and Regulatory Issues*. New York, NY: The Hastings Center.

Lynn, J. (2004) When does quality improvement count as research? Human subject protection and theories of knowledge. *Quality and Safety in Health Care* 13(1): 67–70.

Lynn, J., Baily, M.A., Bottrell, M., Jennings, B., Levine, R.J., Davidoff, F., et al. (2007) The ethics of using quality improvement methods in health care. *Annals of Internal Medicine* 146(9): 666–673.

Miller, F.G. and Emanuel, E.J. (2008) Quality-improvement research and informed consent. *New England Journal of Medicine* 358(8): 765–767.

Nelson, W.A. and Gardent, P.B. (2008) Ethics and healthcare improvement. *Healthcare Executive* Jul/Aug 23(4): 40–41.

Nelson, W.A., Gardent, P.B., Shulman, E., and Splaine, M.E. (2010) Preventing ethics conflicts and improving healthcare quality through system redesign. *Quality and Safety in Healthcare* 19(6): 526–530.

Newhouse, R.P., Pettit, J.C., Poe, S., and Rocco, L. 2006 The slippery slope: Differentiating between quality improvement and research. *Journal of Nursing Administration* 36(4): 211–219.

Nursing and Midwifery Council (2015) *The Code: Professional Standards of Practice and Behaviour for Nurses and Midwives*. Available from: https://www.nmc.org.uk/globalassets/sitedocuments/nmc-publications/nmc-code.pdf (accessed on 1 April 2016).

O'Kane, M.E. (2007) Do patients need to be protected from quality improvement? In: Jennings B, Baily M.A, Bottrell M, Lynn J, editors. *Quality Health Care Quality Improvement: Ethical and Regulatory Issues*. New York, NY: The Hastings Center, pp. 89–99.

Platterborze, L.S., Young-McCaughan, S., King-Letzkus, I., McClinton, A., Halliday A., and Jefferson, TC. (2010) Performance improvement/research advisory panel: A model for determining whether a project is a performance or quality improvement activity or research. *Military Medicine* 175(4): 289–291.

Tapp, L., Elwyn, G., Edwards, A., Holm, S., and Eriksson, T. (2009) Quality improvement in primary care: Ethical issues explored. *International Journal of Healthcare Quality Assurance* 22(1): 8–29.

Taylor, H.A., Pronovost, P.J., and Sugarman, J. (2010) Ethics oversight and quality improvement initiatives. *Quality and Safety in Healthcare* 19(4): 271–274.

Visscher, M., King, A., Nie, A.M., Schaffer, P., Taylor, T., Pruitt, D., Giaccone, M.J., Ashby, M., and Keswani, S. (2013) A quality-improvement collaborative project to reduce pressure ulcers in PICUs. *Pediatrics* 131(6): e1950–e1960.

Wade, D. (2007) Ethics of collecting and using healthcare data. *British Medical Journal* 334(7608): 1330–1331.

Wise, L.C. (2007) Ethical issues surrounding quality improvement activities: A review. *Journal of Nursing Administration* 17(6): 272–278.

Wise, L. (2008) Quality improvement or research? A report from the trenches. *American Journal of Critical Care* 17(2): 98–99.

World Health Organisation (2013) *Ethical Issues in Patient Safety Research: Interpreting Existing Guidance*. Geneva: WHO.

World Medical Association (1964) *Declaration of Helsinki*. Available from: http://www.wma.net/en/30publications/10policies/b3/ (accessed on 1 April 2016).

Wynia M.K. and Kurlander, J.E. (2007) Physician ethics and participation. In: Jennings, B., Baily, M.A., Bottrell, M., Lynn, J., editors. *Quality Health Care Quality Improvement: Ethical and Regulatory Issues*. New York, NY: The Hastings Center, pp. 7–26.

6 Measuring for Healthcare Improvement

Elaine Maxwell

Introduction

Measuring the quality of a product or service is a universal human activity. For example, when assessing apples, people assess the quality of each apple they pick up by judging it on a number of criteria such as colour, texture, smell and taste. This almost subconscious measurement of things gets shared with others and a consensus arises on what constitutes 'good' quality and this becomes the standard or expectation of the quality of an apple.

As Langley et al. (2009) pointed out, in order to know whether an improvement has occurred, it is necessary to ascertain both that a change has happened and that the change has, in fact, been an improvement. Deming (2000) cautioned that it is a mistake to assume that 'if you cannot measure it you cannot improve it,' and it is certainly true that there are many factors in successful quality improvement that are not amenable to quantitative analysis. However, as Berwick (1996) observed, to determine the extent to which a change is an improvement, some form of measurement is required as part of the feedback loop.

Measurement, when thoughtfully conducted, provides information about the nature of the change and what caused it to change, what influenced the change and perhaps even more importantly why a change did not occur and even an indication of the likelihood of an unwanted outcome of the change occurring. This leads to the inevitability that measurement has a key role to play in quality improvement activities. Data collection is almost endemic in healthcare provision which is awash with data, but data alone does not lead to improvement. For improvement there needs to be a clear purpose for the measures, appropriate data collection required to address that purpose and a method of analysis that complements the purpose. Whilst the application of knowledge and improvement is challenging without data, data without knowledge is similarly unlikely to produce improvement.

Deming (2000) emphasised that knowledge of the system and understanding of variation are essential to managing improvement and that this understanding is rarely achieved by single pre- and post-intervention measures or by simply comparing averages which have smoothed out the range of data collected (the variation). Understanding improvement more usually requires study of data over a significant time frame and from a diverse range of sources. Selecting the appropriate measurement plan is an essential part of designing and leading successful improvement projects and involves considering the strengths and weaknesses of different approaches to measuring for improvement.

Objectives

The chapter's objectives are to:

- Provide an overview of measurement and measurement tools
- Explore the differences between measuring for improvement, judgement and research
- Consider the use of metrics and dashboards: performance against self, unintended consequences of spotlighting specific measures and the use of balancing measures
- Understand the use of statistical process control (SPC) charts (including common cause and special cause variations)

Overview of measurement and measurement tools

Knowledge can be developed both through logic and empirical measurement. Traditionally, the latter would be through experimentation with statistical analysis of the data to infer relationships and the extent to which the findings can be generalised. The predominance of experimentation in healthcare research has given statistical inference a primacy as the currency of knowledge with randomised control trials (RCTs) often promoted as the gold standard of a hierarchy of measurement methodologies and this received wisdom spills over into measurement plans for many quality improvement projects in healthcare. However, even within positivist traditions, there is recognition of the limitation of such approaches. Pronovost et al. (2009) argued, for example, that patient harms are often presented as rates, in part for simplicity and in part with the assumption that the rates can be used to compare an organisation's performance against others; however, this can be inappropriate. Pronovost et al. pointed out that attractive as this simplicity sounds, the fact that patient harms should be uncommon (e.g., medication errors with significant consequences) or indeed rare (e.g., wrong site surgery) makes the statistical confidence in the comparisons as low as to make them not only useless but potentially harmful due to the presence of both false positives and false negatives. It is therefore important to understand that there are different measurement tools and that each has a particular purpose and also to select the correct approach to measurement in order to elicit true understanding.

It is often felt that using outcome measures is the best way to measure quality but reaching a consensus definition of how to measure harms can be challenging as evidenced by the debate about how to calculate mortality (a fairly definitive outcome) rates. In the United Kingdom, there are a number of different definitions used to measure hospital mortality rates and the performance of each hospital can vary dramatically according to which definition is used. Following the report into the failings at Mid Staffordshire NHS Foundation Trust in England, where it was suggested that a high number of patients were being coded as receiving palliative care and therefore excluded from hospital mortality figures, Professor Sir Bruce Keogh (Medical Director of the National Health Service [NHS] in England) was asked to conduct a review into the quality of care and treatment provided by hospital trusts with persistently high mortality rates (Keogh 2013). His first task was to identify the trusts with high mortality and he selected 14 trusts on the basis that they had been outliers for the past 2 consecutive years on either the Summary Hospital-Level Mortality Index (SHMI) or the Hospital Standardised Mortality Ratio (HSMR) or both. The SHMI looks at all patients in a hospital and includes all the deaths both in hospital and for 30 days after discharge. It is a ratio of the observed number of deaths to the expected number of deaths. The expected number of deaths is calculated through a risk-adjusted model for each diagnosis group. The HSMR looks at the most serious life-threatening conditions and only includes deaths that take place whilst in the care of the hospital and is risk-adjusted for more factors than the SHMI, most significantly palliative care but also past history of admissions, month of admission and source of admission. It was interesting to note that in Professor Sir Bruce Keogh's review (Keogh 2013), the two different measures gave strikingly different pictures for some of the hospitals with only three identified as having high mortality on both measures. Clearly, improvement projects need a more sophisticated question than simply, 'What is the mortality rate?'

Even when clear questions and inclusion criteria have been agreed, most harms are reported by multiple different staff who have different interpretations of the definitions and different resources available to conduct the measurement. Dixon-Woods et al. (2012) studied the way in which central line infections were measured in intensive care units (ICUs) and then used as part of England's National Patient Safety Agency's 'Matching Michigan' improvement programme (see Chapter 2, Box 2.3). The authors found significant variation both within individual ICUs as to how different staff applied inclusion and exclusion criteria for the programme, and also that systems for collecting the data established in different ICUs were different. Not only that, they also noted differences in how microbiological laboratory support was used and in procedures for presenting data on possible infections. This meant that staff deciding what to report as central line infections were not making decisions in the same way. Even something as apparently clear cut as identifying central line infections turned out to be relatively subjective and reported infection rates reflected localised interpretations rather than a standardised dataset across all ICUs. Crucially, Dixon-Woods et al. concluded that the variation arose not through deliberate manipulation but because counting is as much a social practice as a technical practice.

Measuring purpose

Effective measurement needs prior consideration and a well-developed measurement plan. The first stage of developing the plan is to determine the specific purpose of the measurement, for that will guide the choice from different approaches to data collection and analysis. It is important to understand the implications of the different designs and to carefully consider the assumptions that are being made and the limitations of the conclusions that can be drawn from different data collection and analysis designs. The purpose of each measure should be clearly articulated; this might include providing early warning of hazards, measuring the environmental capacity for improvement, understanding variation in the process or assessing the outcome. The purpose of the measure will inform sampling and inclusion criteria for data collection. Measures must be sensitive enough to measure a modest change and specific enough to link that change to the quality improvement intervention.

Measuring for research

Most healthcare professionals are familiar with quantitative research measurement. This seeks to provide statistical generalisations that can be applied across different settings. Achieving high levels of confidence requires large data sets or power on which to conduct inferential statistical tests. Data is collected in one large test and the aim is to discover new knowledge rather than to explore trends.

Performance measurement

An alternative to measuring for research is the concept of measurement of performance which is drawn from business management principles. This can be a simple measuring of performance against a predetermined target or standard using a relatively simple binary concept of compliance, pass or fail, to determine whether an acceptable standard has been met or not.

The analysis of the data is purely descriptive, with either percentages (e.g., waiting times) or ratios (e.g., mortality rates). Unlike measuring for research, there is no need to generalise and 'just enough' data is often used. This technique is used in clinical audits where 10 records are examined each month as an assurance that the target is not being failed.

In performance measurement, data is often used to benchmark different units or organisations or to rank their quality performance. This provides an opportunity for some competitive motivation amongst units. However, ranking may not identify trends within a specific system and a team or unit that is in the top quartile of a ranking table could be on a downward trend for a significant period of time before it falls below the average and many opportunities for quality improvement may be missed.

More sophisticated performance measures distinguish between three different types of target or standard. The simplest standard is the performance that is currently expected at all times; failure should never occur. The second type of standard is an achievable standard; something that will involve a stretch but is assumed to be achievable within the timescale and available resources. The third type of standard is an aspirational standard, something to aim for without expectation of immediate achievement but which sets a yardstick against which progress can be judged. The choice has important implications; setting an 'expected performance' target may be challenging for some, but others may already be meeting this and may only need to tread water to meet the target and not make any improvement over time. Stretch and aspirational targets are more akin to measuring for improvement as they can be used to measure change rather than compliance and ensure everyone makes an improvement, relative to their starting point.

At organisational level, it is important to understand the variation between units as well as the corporate mean to provide an opportunity to learn from the best performers and to give an indication of what might be possible and to set 'stretch' targets.

Measuring for improvement

Quality improvement measurement seeks to understand a bounded system and recognise the influences within that setting. This means that the measurement plan needs to be set within the context of the local system. Rather than consider performance against targets, quality improvement seeks to learn about the process and the system. Measurement plans are therefore not to generalise to other settings (although evaluation of improvement projects may indeed seek to do this, see Chapter 10) and therefore do not use the inferential statistics, meaning that measurement plans do not require the volume of data that measuring for research requires.

Improvement data is usually presented in time series with as little reduction to summarised data as possible. As improvement projects progress and there is increasing understanding of the process, interventions may change and data definitions may expand. A good example of this is adverse events, where the definition of preventable adverse event has changed steadily over the last 10 years and is likely to continue to expand. Using a time series chart, it is possible to annotate changes to definitions, changed interventions and their consequences. Rather than being a limitation of the measurement plan, the dynamic development of criteria indicates the increasing maturity of a quality improvement management system and the development of a learning organisation.

Learning organisations

Argyris and Schön (1978) described two levels of organisational learning. First there is single-loop learning, where compliance with explicit practices, policies and norms of behaviour is measured and this is akin to performance measurement. Learning from the measures involves detecting and correcting deviations and variances from these standards and seeks to find a better way to conduct the same process. Single-loop learning helps stable systems with little variation to achieve high levels of consistency and is useful for maintaining a steady state. Improvement is achieved by increasing the reliability of a process that is fit for purpose.

At times, the process design is not fit for the purpose and improvement requires change. Argris and Schön suggest that this is achieved through double-loop learning, which looks at the performance and then goes on a step further and asks questions about the process itself. Double-loop learning not only measures what is being done in practice but also whether the processes are appropriate and whether a different process might provide better results.

Indicators and balancing measures

Most healthcare providers collect a defined set of data that are then used as proxies for the overall level of quality. The chosen measures are often called metrics or key performance indicators (KPIs) and are selected because they are assumed to represent wider processes and systems. This has the advantage of providing ongoing monitoring, often as a visual dashboard display. Understanding the purpose of the measures is key to making this approach successful. Began and Hood (2006) cautioned against the unintended consequences of focusing on proxy measures, concluding that what is measured becomes what matters. The challenge is that, spotlighting certain measures may lead to attention being focused on the processes they reflect at the expense of others. Whilst it is important for car drivers to measure fuel levels, they also need to monitor oil levels and the air pressure of their tyres. Fuel levels alone, although important, will not tell them anything about oil or air pressure and the short-term advantage of focusing on fuel but not tyre pressure might be a dangerous choice in the long term.

In a similar manner, ensuring timely access to care is an important element of high-quality care, but it is not the only element. If the focus on measuring the number of people treated and discharged from emergency departments within 4 hours is not balanced by other measures, the consequence might be that attention is paid solely to the throughput. The consequence of this might be to increase the numbers of patients being admitted to hospital to avoid breaching the performance target. An unintended consequence of this might be the need to discharge patients (without any regards to the relative needs of those being admitted and those being discharged) more quickly in order to free up space for the increased admissions. Performance against the simple 4-hour wait target will not pick up the implications further down the system and so any adverse or unintentional consequence may go unremarked. Measurement plans should include balancing measures that indicate the impact on other parts of the system of acting to meet a single target.

Focusing on a single part of the system can also inhibit the search for the improvements that will lead to compliance with that target. In order to truly understand how to improve access, data that clearly describes the whole system is needed. If an emergency department is failing to meet the waiting time target for patients to be seen and discharged, there are a range of things that might be done to improve the situation. There could be an increase in the number of staff to ensure that there are no delays in the consultation, it might be decided to divert less acute patients to a minor injury or primary care service or there might be a change to the roles of existing staff and advanced practitioners might see and treat patients, leaving medical staff to manage the critically ill. Choosing the right solution depends on fully understanding the nature of the problem and choosing the wrong intervention might not only fail to improve performance, it might cause problems elsewhere (critically ill patients might be inadvertently directed to minor injury units) and potentially increase costs for no gain.

Mannion and Goddard (2002) caution against inferring too much from indicators and running the risk of mistakenly classifying either poor performance (type I errors) or providing false assurance (type II errors). Indicators are just that: prompts for further investigation which will involve different measurement approaches.

Process mapping

Process mapping is a technique to understand the flow of activity between the constituent parts of the process. Indicators can provide alerts that a process is not performing as desired but process maps are needed to describe in detail what is happening within the process: which part(s) of the process could be improved to improve the performance of the whole. Process mapping often involves visual representation of the sequence of activities and is used extensively within LEAN methods to identify which activities are slowing down the flow and/or are failing to add any value to the process. For example, a process-mapping exercise might find that a patient is seen at home by a number of different healthcare professionals, each of whom keeps his or her own records and who asks the patient the same questions. This is a result of the process design and there is no independent added value of the separate records. The failure to share records means that communication between the healthcare professionals is delayed and the patient has to wait for services. Moving to electronic records would remove the wasted time, the irritation to the patient of having to repeat the same information and add value by allowing each professional to see the other's entries and make swift decisions and intervene promptly.

Process mapping can be used to explore simple tasks, such as record keeping or can be used to map patient journeys or pathways through a whole care episode. They can also be used to understand business processes, such as managing referrals and waiting lists.

To map a process, it is important to gain the contribution of people looking at the process from different angles, including administrators, porters, estate staff as well as health professionals and probably, most importantly, patients. As an example, Figure 6.1 portrays the process of getting an image of a suspected fractured ankle for a patient presenting at an emergency department. The complexity of processes can be seen through mapping the number of steps taken to obtain a radiological image for a suspected simple fracture; there are 18 steps and three different departments involved.

What to measure?

Vincent et al. (2013) synthesised the academic literature to produce a framework for measuring patient safety, the principles of which could equally apply to quality improvement more widely. They identified the following five domains, which they suggest together would provide a comprehensive measurement and monitoring system:

1 **Past performance:** Measuring past performance gives a base indication of the direction of travel and of the system outcomes.
2 **System and process reliability:** Regardless of the outcomes (which may be in spite of rather than because of the design, chance having a material impact), measuring whether the system and the processes reliably perform as intended.
3 **Current performance:** The real-time performance.
4 **Preparedness:** Drawing on the High Reliability Organisation literature, measuring the capacity to anticipate and respond to threats to quality.
5 **Learning and improving:** Tracking the organisation's learning and its capacity for improvement.

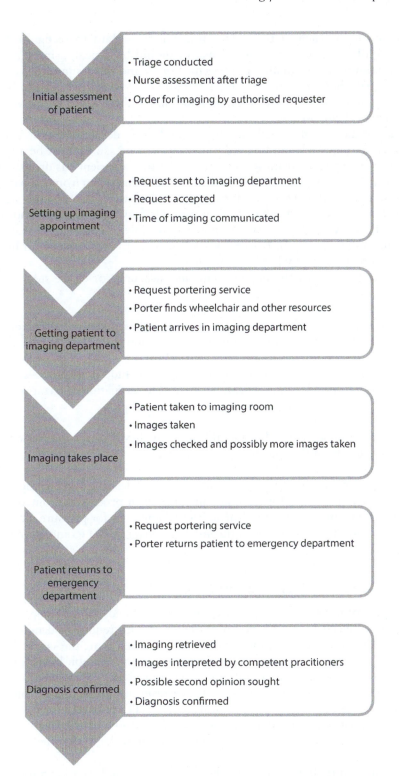

Figure 6.1 Mapping the process of getting an image of a suspected fractured ankle in a person pre-senting at an emergency department.

In order to address each of these domains, it is important to recognise the dynamic, iterative nature of improvement work. Measures should be logical, using the best evidence available and relevant to the quality improvement goal and the assumptions about how the improvement goal (the change to be demonstrated) will be achieved need to be articulated. Measurement is an important part of testing and refining these assumptions and of adapting evidence to the local circumstances.

The impact of measurement will only be as good as its design. Without a well-reasoned plan, the measures may lack validity and reliability. The measures must be a true reflection of the goal. For example, if a team want to know whether a patient has drunk enough fluids, they might assume that measuring how much water has been taken from the patient's bedside jug will answer the question. However, it may be that the patient has used this water for other purposes, such as cleaning his teeth or rinsing cups. He may have used it to moisten a flannel or to top up a flower vase. What seems at first to be an obvious and simple way of collecting data about the amount a patient has drunk now appears to be a measure of how much has been used but not necessarily what has been drunk.

Measures can be of either the impact (outcome measures) or of the steps taken towards the outcome (process):

- **Process measures** are often described as leading indicators as they provide information upstream about what leads to the outcomes. Breaking the whole process down into the component steps and describing their relationship to the intended outcome will help to identify the appropriate measures and is likely to include both processes and outcome measures. Monitoring leading indicators can lead to mitigation of hazards and unwanted outcomes.

- **Outcome measures** are called lagging indicators as they describe the consequences of the process: the impact of the changes.

Quality improvement is dependent on monitoring both leading and lagging measures. The safety thermometer (Box 6.1), for example, includes both process and outcomes measures, although not both related to the same harm. It uses outcomes for pressure ulcers (number of pressure ulcers) and process for venous thromboembolism (VTE) (completion of a VTE risk assessment).

Determining the type of data for measurement

Once the purpose of measuring has been explored and defined, the next step is to ensure that the data which is collected is a reflection of the concept. This requires a detailed specification of what is included or excluded in the data collection. When using the safety thermometer it is important to consider: what is a pressure ulcer? Does it include non-blanching erythema of intact skin or does it require more significant tissue injury? Does it include sores on ears and nostrils? Failure to establish this at the outset may result in different data collectors including different things. Similarly, the process measure for VTEs is the completion of a VTE risk assessment and might be restricted to the risk assessment protocol or it might be expanded to the decision-making as a result of the assessment or even evidence that the proposed actions were indeed taken.

Where it is difficult to directly measure the improvement under consideration, an option is to collect proxy data: data that does not directly measure but appears to coexist or correlate to the improvement goal and gives an indication of the desired change. An example might be

Box 6.1 The safety thermometer

The safety thermometer was developed in response to the Department of Health in England's Quality, Innovation, Productivity and Prevention (QIPP) programme. The QIPP's safety work stream focused on four high-volume harms (safety outcomes): pressure ulcers, falls, urinary tract infection (UTI) in patients with catheters and venous thromboembolism (VTE), which were estimated to affect over 200,000 people a year and cost £430 million in England (Power et al. 2012). Measurement had been dependent on voluntary reporting of adverse incidents or labour intensive reviews of medical records. The safety thermometer counts the percentage of patients on a single day each month who have not experienced any of the four identified harms and uses this as a proxy for 'harm free care'. The safety thermometer was designed to be a pragmatic tool, and the authors suggest that in the same way that recording increased temperature does not diagnose the problem but signals a need for further investigation, data from the safety thermometer can indicate a need for more detailed exploration of performance in relation to safety.

The operating framework for the National Health Service (NHS) in England 2012/13 (Department of Health 2011) included the safety thermometer as part of the Commissioning for Quality and Innovation (CQUIN) scheme to incentivise all English providers of NHS care to use the safety thermometer. NHS trusts report the safety thermometer findings as part of their operational management reports and Illingworth (2015) reported that over five million patients have been surveyed with the percentage of people in hospital without any of the four harms rising from 91% in July 2012 to 93.7% in February 2015.

the extent to which patients feel safe during healthcare interventions; whilst this is hard to directly measure, the number of complaints made might be used as a proxy. Proxy measures cannot give absolute measures but can show trends and indicate whether there is likely to be an increase or decrease in the concept under consideration. Heeding Deming's advice to appreciate the whole system, improvement projects should include measures from a range of sources, process and outcome, direct and proxy which, when triangulated, will also give a more comprehensive picture of the performance of the whole system.

Data can be collected for each quality improvement or it may be possible to conduct secondary analysis of existing data that has been collected for some other purpose. There are advantages and disadvantages of both approaches. Using existing data is convenient, cheap and does not burden staff with additional work; however, the choice of inclusion and exclusion criteria used in the data collection may not perfectly match those of the improvement project. For example, measuring infection rates by monitoring the prescription of antibiotics is easy and convenient but will not include infections that for whatever reason were not treated pharmaceutically. On the other hand, setting up new systems can lead to issues of reliability if staff are not committed to the project and consider this data to be a low priority in their work.

How to analyse quality improvement measures

Data is not an end in itself but a tool to understand processes that influence quality. Data interpretation is rarely self-evident and data only becomes useful through analysis. As Langley et al. (2009) advised, it is important to understand not only when has a change occurred but also whether that change is an improvement. It is also important to know whether that improvement had anything to do with the improvement interventions. These questions each require different data analysis methods.

Performance data is usually presented in tabular form or grouped into categories (such as the Red, Amber, Green 'RAG' rating system) to 'smooth' large amounts of data into manageable chunks thus avoiding information overload. This inevitably means a loss of detail. Improvement data should, on the other hand, keep as much detail as possible and tell a story that guides the reader through the improvement process journey. Improvement is an internal change and measuring improvement involves comparing own performance over time; measuring improvement is therefore a matter of looking for trends and for links between the trend and specific improvement processes. Improvement often follows an S-shaped rather than a linear journey, with early success through the gains from 'low hanging fruits' or simple improvements, followed by a plateau until a breakthrough in understanding of more complex issues occurs and then finally, an incremental improvement towards the aspirational goal.

Run charts and Statistical Process Control (SPC) charts

Box 6.2 provides definitions of terms used in this section.

One way to measure change is to display data on a run chart or time series which show data over time (see example Figure 6.2). Run charts use the middle value (median) as a benchmark and data analysis is based on whether points are above or below that middle value. No account is taken of the relative distances from the median; only whether a value is above or below and so run charts show change but are not sensitive in detecting the size of any variation.

Shewhart (1939) described two different patterns of variation, controlled (or common cause) and uncontrolled (special cause), that could be determined statistically and displayed on charts that would differentiate between them. Shewhart's contribution to the history of quality improvement is discussed in Chapter 1. His SPC charts use probability testing and vary according to the assumptions of data distribution. However, in most cases, a normal distribution is assumed and SPC charts calculate plus or minus three standard deviations from the mean. Like all statistical tests, the confidence is dependent on the power of the calculation and too few data points may give false positives and negatives. However, with sufficient data, 95% of the range variation is predicted and the extremes of this range are described as control limits, hence the charts are called control charts. The control limits define extent

---

Box 6.2 Definitions relevant to analysing data in improvement

Mean: The arithmetical mean is the calculation of the sum of all the individual values divided by the total number of values. The mean is an artificial value and may not reflect any single actual observed value.

Median: The middle value of all the observed values.

Normal distribution: Normal (or Gaussian) distribution of data is a stable pattern of data distribution that resembles a bell and is the basis for a number of statistical tests. Where data is not distributed in this pattern, those statistical tests are not appropriate.

Standard deviation: Means and medians do not indicate the range of variation or deviance in the data observed. Standard deviation is a statistical test showing the distance from the mean of the most different values observed.

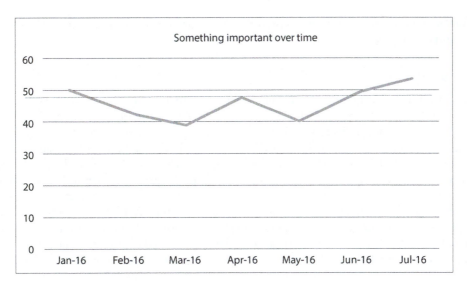

Figure 6.2 Example of a run chart.

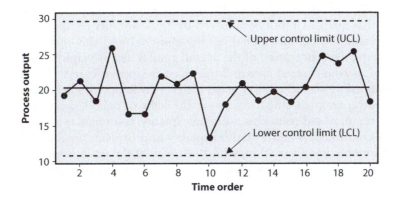

Figure 6.3 Example of how apparent improvement is a highly variable process.

of variation that might be anticipated in a given process and said to be common to the process. Data points that fall within the control limit are seen to be common to the process or 'common cause' variation. Any data that falls outside the control limits raises the question of whether there was a special cause of the variation, something external to the process. Figure 6.3 displays how apparent improvement is a highly variable process.

As well as showing the nature of the variation, SPC charts allow analysis of two further important but different measures. They can measure the direction of travel by tracking the mean of all the data. This of course varies but when there are seven data points in the same direction outside the existing mean, it is reasonable to assume that there has been a consistent and stepwise change and to reset the mean of the chart and the control limits. This is often called a 'breakthrough'.

Using the mean and standard deviations means that the reliability of performance can also be monitored. Even with a mean travelling in the right direction, the range can be large indicating that different patients or different time periods can experience very different performances. Whilst changes to the mean are often afforded high attention (e.g., a 10% reduction in a given harm), this can mask a very variable process and the most significant quality improvement gains are often to be found in making care more consistent and reliable, whilst retaining the same mean.

Managing variation

The data shows the range of variation but the management of the variation is dependent on the interpretation of the data. An SPC chart with data that falls within the predicted range (the control limits) does not indicate whether the process is good, bad or indifferent, merely that it is stable or, as Shewhart described it, in statistical control. Managing variation requires a diagnosis of the nature of the variation and whether the variation is inherent in the process design or caused by some external factor. Changing the design of a process when in fact special cause (external cause) variation has occurred will at best be useless and at worst, may cause system-related performance to deteriorate. What is required is to explore the system and see what the external factors are and how they might be mitigated. If the variation is within the predicted (control) limits, that is to say common cause variation, the goal is to reduce the range of variation: to increase the reliability so that the performance is consistent in different circumstances.

Intentional and unintentional variation

It is often said that quality is achieved through the elimination of variation; on the other hand, it is said that quality cannot be achieved by a one-size-fits-all approach. Variation can be desirable or undesirable, intentional or unintentional and this distinction can only be made through careful consideration of the overall goal. A key principle of modern healthcare is individualised, person-centred care and this must mean that care will vary between people as their personal as well as clinical needs differ. This happens when expert professionals consciously make context-specific decisions in the light of complex variables that may not be included in standardised protocols, although quality assurance is needed to ensure that the variation was justified. A better goal for quality improvement might be the reduction or elimination of *unintentional* variation, whilst celebrating the intentional variation that calibrates the process to meet local conditions and individual patient's needs.

Historic or real-time data

Quality reports often feature post hoc data, anything between 1 month and 1 year in arrears. This is useful for performance evaluation and for quality assurance but does not provide the real-time data needed during the process of improvement. Real-time quality measures anticipate hazards that might threaten the implementation and embedding of the change. Improvement projects need to be alerted to these hazards so as to manage them early before they become larger challenges. This is akin to the speed, fuel and oil indicators on a car dashboard that give the driver real-time information of how the car is performing. The driver can use this information to predict whether there are imminent risks and decide whether to take any direct action to avoid them. Giving healthcare professionals access to real-time performance data can help them to intentionally vary their actions to safeguard the outcomes, rather than follow a standard process at the expense of the outcome.

Data visualisation

The complexity of healthcare systems means, it is more likely that improvement is a case of two steps forward, one step backward. Interpretation needs to be mindful of subtle patterns within a mass of confusing data, and this can sometimes be more readily observed through visualisation than through numerical tables. One of the early proponents of data visualisation in healthcare was Florence Nightingale who produced her 'Diagram of the Causes of Mortality in the Army' in the East in late 1858 (see Figure 1.1 in Chapter 1). Producing a visual display clearly demonstrated that most of the British soldiers who died during the Crimean War died of sickness rather than of wounds or other causes and helped her to focus improvement attention to sanitation and hygiene as a way of reducing deaths (Nightingale 1858).

More recently, safety crosses have been used to demonstrate the frequency of adverse events in given areas, such as pressure ulcer incidence. The cross has 31 boxes, each representing a day of the month and boxes that are left empty are those when no pressure ulcer was found, whilst days that have been shaded in show new pressure ulcers identified on that day (see Figure 6.4). Whilst this does not contain the sophistication of an SPC chart, it is an effective way of raising awareness of an issue and triggering an appetite for further investigation.

Visualisation can be useful to determine the relative priorities for improvement. In the 1950s, Juran suggested the 80/20 principle, based on the Italian economist Pareto who showed that approximately 80% of the land in Italy was owned by 20% of the population and observed that 20% of the peapods in his garden contained 80% of the peas. Juran coined the phrase 'Pareto principle' to describe how a small number of factors cause a large number of challenges and that quality improvement efforts are best directed to establish these factors, thereby determining the priority area to focus effort and the order in which to tackle them (Sanders 1987). A Pareto diagram is a bar chart with the possible areas for improvement displayed in descending order according to the size of the impact. The cumulative impact is plotted on a line to show the combined impact of two or more factors.

Figure 6.5 portrays a hypothetical situation in which most of the problems in delivering medicines on time come from issues around generic versus trade names or the drug being out of stock. Quality improvement projects that focus on these areas will have the most impact. Improvement projects that focus on the prescriber's writing will have only marginal impact on the delivery of medicines.

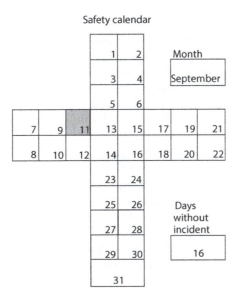

Figure 6.4 Safety cross.

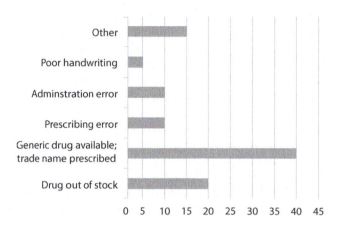

Figure 6.5 Causes of missed medications in hospitals by percentage of all.

Measuring the context for quality improvement, culture and climate

The importance of context in quality improvement, especially around cultures and their impact on change is gaining increasing attention and is explored in detail in Chapter 2. In early work on this subject, Pettigrew et al. (1992) studied changes in the NHS during the 1980s and found that success was dependent on the interplay of the context, the process and the content of change together with the leaders' skill in regulating the relations amongst the three. Pettigrew concluded that a change cannot be understood as an entity in itself, devoid of its context and the process of implementation. More recently, Fan et al. (2016) have shown that post-operative infection rates in the state of Minnesota were strongly associated with safety culture scores and in particular, organisational feedback and communication related to errors. Measuring culture is therefore likely to be a useful tool in quality improvement.

Culture is a broad term covering a number of different concepts, although it commonly includes having a sense of common purpose and teamwork. The UK Health and Safety Executive (2005) draw a distinction between three different concepts of culture. First there is the behavioural aspect (i.e., what people do), second the structural aspects (i.e., what resources the organisation has) and finally the concept of climate which refers to the psychological characteristics of employees (i.e., how people feel). This distinction is important as it illustrates a potential difference between values and attitudes (intentions) and actual behaviours in the workplace.

Weiner (2009) suggested that perceptions can be subdivided into commitment to a behaviour or change and belief that the change of behaviour will be effective. Organisational readiness for improvement will be dependent on high levels of both. This echoes Festinger (1957), who described the situation where people experience conflict between their values and their behaviours, termed 'cognitive dissonance' and suggests that this is an untenable position, which the human mind seeks to resolve as soon as possible. Resolution is achieved by changing either the values or the behaviours. Changing learned (or socialised) behaviours is difficult and if not achieved, the values are altered to avoid cognitive dissonance. The theory has been used to explain the attitudes of people who continue to display risky health behaviours such as smoking, despite clear motivation to be healthy. Whilst it does not explain the behaviour completely, cognitive dissonance theory does imply that structural conditions are as important for improvement as personal motivation.

It therefore follows that measuring the behavioural and situational aspects of culture may reveal different information about what is shaping an organisation than measuring attitudes and perceptions. Many of the tools currently used for assessing the culture of an organisation are standardised surveys of staff or users' perception ratings (values and attitudes) and their limitations in measuring culture are acknowledged by describing them as measuring climate rather than culture. A number of academics studying improvement use ethnographic methods to elicit structural and behavioural aspects, for example Leslie et al. (2014) (see Chapter 2).

Patient/service user role in measuring quality

Measuring the patient's or consumer's experience of care is well established within health-care and with the increasing focus on co-production, attention is increasingly being paid to engaging them in a more active contribution to assessing quality. A roundtable on involving patients in safety held in 2013 by the Health Foundation concluded that:

> The patient is the single most important safety barometer and the issues they raise can be an early warning to a later risk. The unhelpful distinction that has traditionally been made between care and treatment has led to a view that some complaints are 'only about care', leaving staff unable to understand the risks to safety from patient feedback.
>
> (Health Foundation 2013, p. 2)

Whilst patients may not be able to assess the technical aspects of clinical care, they are often the only people to have an appreciation of the whole system of their care and as a result, they bring a different lens to the process. Scott et al. (2011) demonstrated how patients often have different perceptions of safety from healthcare professionals. Whereas healthcare professionals focus on technical processes and physical outcomes such as medication issues, falls and healthcare-acquired infections, patients perceive social factors such as communication, responsiveness and trust to be as important as the clinical hazards identified by healthcare professionals. This view appears to be supported by Weissman et al. (2008) who suggest that patients can identify safety issues that staff may not notice or might not be willing or able to report. Chapter 4 focuses on service user involvement in improvement in detail.

Conclusion

Measurement is a key activity for quality improvement and requires as much consideration as designing interventions. Measurement of the situation prior to an improvement project should inform the setting of the improvement goal and can identify the appropriate process and the efforts that are likely to produce the most benefit. Measures are also necessary to monitor the progress of the improvement and pick up any early warnings of hazards that might threaten the improvement goal as well as the outcome.

The importance of measurement should be acknowledged at the beginning of any project and a measurement plan devised with due regard to the different purposes of measurement. Clarity of purpose will direct the data collection and data analysis methods that will support the successful implementation of the improvement project.

References

Argyris, C. and Schön, D.A. (1978) *Organizational Learning: A Theory of Action Perspective*. Reading, MA: Addison-Wesley.

Began, G. and Hood, C. (2006) What's measured is what matters: Targets and gaming in the English public health care system. *Public Administration* 84(3): 517–538.

Berwick, D.M. (1996) A primer on leading the improvement of systems. *BMJ: British Medical Journal* 312(7031): 619.

Deming, W. (2000) *The New Economics: For Industry, Government, Education*. Cambridge, MA: Massachusetts Institute of Technology Press.

Department of Health (2011) *NHS Operating Framework for 2012/13*. London: DH. Available from: https://www.gov.uk/government/uploads/system/uploads/attachment_data/file/216590/dh_131 428.pdf (accessed on 28 April 2016).

Dixon-Woods, M., Leslie, M., Bion, J., and Tarrant, C. (2012) What counts? An ethnographic study of infection data reported to a patient safety program. *Milbank Quarterly* 90(3): 548–591.

Fan, C., Pawlik, T., Daniels, T., Vernon, N., Banks, K., Westby, P., Wick, E., Sexton, J., and Makary, M. (2016) Association of safety culture with surgical site infection outcomes. *Journal of the American College of Surgeons* 222(2): 122–128.

Festinger, L. (1957) *A Theory of Cognitive Dissonance*. Stanford, CA: Stanford University Press.

Health and Safety Executive (2005) *A Review of Safety Culture and Safety Climate Literature for the Development of the Safety Culture Inspection Toolkit*. Available from: http://www.hse.gov.uk/research/rrpdf/rr367.pdf (accessed on 26 August 2016).

Health Foundation (2013) *Involving People in Safety: A Summary of Learning from a Health Foundation Roundtable*. London: Health Foundation.

Illingworth, J. (2015) *Is the NHS Getting Safer?* London: Health Foundation.

Keogh, B. (2013) *Review into the Quality of Care and Treatment Provided by 14 Hospital Trusts in England: Overview Report*. Available from: http://www.nhs.uk/NHSEngland/bruce-keogh-review/Documents/outcomes/keogh-review-final-report.pdf (accessed on 28 April 2016).

Langley, G., Moen, R., Nolan, K., Nolan, T., Norman, C., and Provost, L. (2009) *The Improvement Guide: A Practical Approach to Enhancing Organizational Performance*. San Francisco, CA: John Wiley & Sons.

Leslie, M., Paradis, E., Gropper, M.A., Reeves, S., and Kitto, S. (2014) Applying ethnography to the study of context in healthcare quality and safety. *BMJ Quality and Safety* 23(2): 99–105.

Mannion, R. and Goddard, M. (2002) Performance measurement and improvement in health care. *Applied Health Economics and Health Policy* 1(1): 13–23.

Nightingale, F. (1858) *Notes on Matters Affecting the Health, Efficiency, and Hospital Administration of the British Army: Founded Chiefly on the Experience of the Late War*. Presented by Request to the Secretary of State for War. London: Harrison and Sons.

Pettigrew, A., Ferlie, E., and McKee, L. (1992) Shaping strategic change– The case of the NHS in the 1980s. *Public Money and Management* 12(3): 27–31.

Power, M., Stewart, K., and Brotherton, A. (2012) What is the NHS Safety Thermometer? *Clinical Risk* 18(5): 163–169.

Pronovost, P.J., Goeschel, C.A., Marsteller, J.A., Sexton, J.B., Pham, J.C., and Berenholtz, S.M. (2009) Framework for patient safety research and improvement. *Circulation* 119(2): 330–337.

Sanders, R. (1987) The Pareto principle: Its use and abuse. *Journal of Services Marketing* 1(2): 37–40.

Scott, J., Dawson, P., and Jones, D. (2012) Do older patients' perceptions of safety highlight barriers that could make their care safer during organisational care transfers? *BMJ Quality and Safety* 21(2): 112–117.

Shewhart, W. (1939) *Statistical Method from the Viewpoint of Quality Control*. Washington, DC: Graduate School of the Department of Agriculture.

Vincent, C., Burnett, S., and Carthey, J. (2013) *The Measurement and Monitoring of Safety*. London: Health Foundation.

Weiner, B.J. (2009) A theory of organizational readiness for change. *Implement Science* 4(1): 67.

Weissman, J., Schneider, E., and Weingart, S. (2008) Comparing patient-reported hospital adverse events with medical record review: Do patients know something that hospitals do not? *Annals of Internal Medicine* 149: 100–108.

7 High Reliability Organisations: Making Care Safer through Reliability and Resilience

Mark Sujan

Introduction

This chapter provides an overview of some of the key lessons from the theory of industrial High Reliability Organisations (HROs) that might be applied in healthcare in order to improve the safety of care delivered to patients. HROs have been described as organisations that manage to have few or no significant accidents even though they operate complex technology in highly hazardous environments, such as aircraft carriers and nuclear power plants (La Porte 1996).

Patient safety is an area of significant public concern. In the United Kingdom, there has been much media coverage of the findings of the Public Inquiry into the failings at Mid Staffordshire NHS Foundation Trust. The report suggests that between 2005 and 2009 as many as 1200 patients died needlessly as a result of inadequate and often appalling standards of care (Francis 2013). Research undertaken in different countries and different health systems has provided ample evidence that patients around the world are suffering preventable adverse events (Vincent et al. 2001; Davis et al. 2002; Baker et al. 2004; de Vries et al. 2008; Thomas et al. 2000; Brennan et al. 1991). Adverse events cause unnecessary suffering and they also have significant financial implications resulting from additional bed days and extended care requirements of patients, as well as from increased insurance and litigation costs (Vincent et al. 2001; Ovretveit 2009).

In order to improve patient safety, and to reduce the number of adverse events, healthcare organisations have been encouraged to consider lessons about safety management practices in safety-critical industries (Department of Health 2000; Kohn et al. 2000). For example, commercial aviation is considered an ultra-safe industry and there have been frequent attempts to transfer some of the tools, methods and approaches from this industry to healthcare. Examples include the introduction of incident reporting systems (Barach and Small 2000) and the adoption of aviation-style checklists to manage safety-critical tasks, such as the World Health Organisation (WHO) surgical safety checklist (Haynes et al. 2009). Learning from industry is a reasonable suggestion (Kapur et al. 2016), but the successful transfer of lessons from industry to healthcare often proves to be challenging in practice (Sujan et al. 2016; Clay-Williams and Colligan 2015). When transferring and applying lessons from industry to healthcare it is important to understand the underlying theory, the benefits and the limitations of tools and methods within their original industrial context (Sutcliffe et al. 2016).

The aim of this chapter is to provide a brief overview of the theory of HROs as developed in industrial contexts, and based on this, to identify some lessons that might be helpful in

texts to make the delivery of care both more reliable and safer. The next sec-
the key characteristics of industrial HROs. The following three sections then
1 lessons from the theory of HROs for enhancing the reliability of care, for
livery of care more resilient, and for organisational learning. A summary of the
icludes the chapter.

Objectives

The chapter's objectives are to:

- Provide an overview of the theory of High Reliability Organisations
- Introduce principles of risk analysis and risk control for enhancing reliability
- Highlight the importance of performance variability for enhancing resilience
- Discuss the role of organisational learning for sustaining progress with patient safety

Theory of High Reliability Organisations (HROs)

The importance of studying what goes well

Traditionally, organisations and systems aim to learn from what goes wrong (Hollnagel 2014), for example by analysing aviation accidents or by investigating the accidental release of toxic materials from chemical processing plants. The aim of learning from such extraordinary catastrophes is to prevent similar events from recurring (Sujan and Furniss 2015). In the 1980s, a group of researchers at the University of California, Berkeley, suggested that novel insights into safety management and improved safety performance might be developed by studying organisations that had successfully avoided disaster despite operating with complex technology in hazardous situations. The group studied in depth the safety management activities and safety behaviours of three types of organisations with an outstanding safety record – the U.S. air traffic control system, a company operating a nuclear power plant and an electricity distribution system, and the U.S. Navy's operation of aircraft carriers (La Porte and Consolini 1998; Roberts 1990, 1993). The basic premise of the resulting theory of HROs is that there are processes, systems and behaviours that can be put in place that enable organisations operating complex technology in hazardous conditions to prevent and recover from errors in order to maintain an exceptional safety record over long periods of time. In order to understand what these processes, systems and behaviours are, and how they can be sustained in practice, it is necessary to study not only how organisations fail, but also how they succeed to avert disaster on a daily basis, that is to study their ordinary, everyday performance (Sujan et al. 2016; Hollnagel 2014b).

A model of HROs – Mindful organising

The original empirical research did not set out explicitly to study HROs. This term was coined during the research, and there have been numerous definitions of what an HRO might look like. This has not been without controversy, and it has been suggested that it is actually not possible to identify objectively whether an organisation is, or is not, an HRO (Hopkins 2007, 2014). Based on the HRO research, Weick and colleagues developed a model of what they then referred to as 'mindful organisation' (Weick and Sutcliffe 2007). This model describes a number of characteristics and behaviours that organisations should aspire to in order to manage safety. The model can be thought of as an ideal rather than as something concrete against which organisations can be measured (Hopkins 2007). The five organisational characteristics and behaviours are (Weick and Sutcliffe 2007): (1) preoccupation with failures, (2) reluctance to simplify, (3) sesitivity to operations, (4) commitment to resilience and (5) deference to expertise. These are discussed in turn in the following, and then put into a healthcare context in the subsequent sections.

Preoccupation with failure

A good past safety track record might lead to complacency, the diversion of resources for reasons of efficiency, and a reluctance to report and to acknowledge evidence that might call the good performance into question. HROs are preoccupied with failure because they seek out evidence of even small errors, and they treat these as potential precursors to larger failures and disaster. They encourage active reporting and speaking up by frontline staff, and they ensure that as an organisation they have the capacity to listen and to act on such concerns. Often, these errors and early warning signs are, in fact, innocent and without further consequence, but staff are congratulated for reporting these rather than reprimanded for wasting time or causing unnecessary problems.

Reluctance to simplify

In order to manage an organisation in a complex environment one has to simplify and get on with things. However, simplification means discarding some information as noise in favour of other more salient aspects and this bears the risk of discarding the wrong information. HROs breed a reluctance to simplify explanations by fostering a culture of diverse viewpoints and of constructive criticism. They avoid simplistic interpretations of failures such as labelling them human errors. HROs invest in diversity, and they create an infrastructure that provides resource to investigate and pursue potential problems proactively and more widely.

Sensitivity to operations

HROs are sensitive to operations by being attentive to the experience of frontline staff. They recognise that in their complex operating environment, frontline staff have to adapt to the situations on the ground. Managers in HROs encourage staff to report their concerns and to speak up about any errors, safety problems or other potential sources of failure. HROs recognise that a culture of fear might disable the necessary flow of information and prevent the organisation from functioning and adapting effectively.

Commitment to resilience

HROs are not error free, but they are able to deal with errors and contain their consequences before they can lead to actual failures. This is achieved through a commitment to resilience, which, in practice, requires investment in systems, processes and people to provide redundancy and overlap in order to recover from errors. Critical infrastructure might be duplicated, alternative ways of achieving goals are planned and designed, and staff are trained to deal with failures and to improvise novel ways of working and workarounds to existing problems.

Deference to expertise

In time-critical situations, decisions are delegated to the people with the greatest level of relevant expertise, rather than to the member of staff with the highest level of formal authority.

This enables HROs to act quickly in changing and challenging environments. HROs also cultivate a culture of listening to expertise, for example in situations that are not time-critical, but where technical experts might raise concerns. In these situations, staff can abort missions or escalate their concerns irrespective of their ranking in the organisational hierarchy.

Steps towards becoming an HRO

The model of mindful organising sets out an ideal set of characteristics and behaviours to which organisations can aspire. It is unlikely, or even unrealistic, that an organisation can simply adopt these principles from one moment to another across all of its operations in a uniform manner. The more likely scenario is that organisations will have to go through a journey towards becoming an HRO, and this journey might be faster in some areas, and slower and more cumbersome in other areas of an organisation (Carroll and Rudolph 2006). Certain aspects might be more developed in one area, whilst other aspects are better implemented elsewhere.

The model of mindful organising is closely linked to issues of reliability and managing known risks on the one hand, and to resilience and adaptive capacity to deal with changes and surprises on the other hand. These two abilities – to control known risks and to adapt to changes – are underpinned by a third ability, which is the ability to continuously learn and evolve as an organisation.

Enhancing reliability – Risk analysis and risk control

The need for reliable care processes

There is plenty of evidence to suggest that care processes are generally not delivered reliably. In the area of medicines management and prescribing, studies have suggested that prescribing errors occur in 1.5%–9.2% of hospital medication orders (Vincent et al. 2009). This wide range of figures is due to differences in settings, definitions and data collection methods. A median error rate of 7% was reported in an international systematic review of prescribing errors in handwritten medication orders for hospital inpatients (Lewis et al. 2009). A major study in the United States found that patients received scientifically recommended care in only 55% of the cases (McGlynn et al. 2003). However, there were significant differences depending on the condition considered. For example, patients received 78.7% of recommended care for senile cataract in contrast to as little as 10.5% for alcohol dependence. This evidence suggests that there is large variation in the reliability of different care processes, and that, overall, care processes have a significant failure rate that can be improved upon.

Identifying and controlling risks

In order to improve the reliability of processes, organisations usually attempt to exert greater managerial control over how care is delivered (Carroll and Rudolph 2006). This can often be in the form of simplification and standardisation of processes, for example through the use of process mapping (Leonard et al. 2004), LEAN methodologies (Jones and Mitchell 2006; Womack et al. 1990) and the introduction of care bundles (Pronovost et al. 2006).

Another frequently recommended approach is the use of a method called failure mode and effects analysis (FMEA) (DeRosier et al. 2002). FMEA is a proactive, inductive, bottom-up approach for analysing processes in order to identify and to evaluate the main vulnerabilities and the potential for failures. Like process mapping, FMEA is carried out in a multi-disciplinary group setting in order to ensure that different perspectives are considered. FMEA often starts with a process map and then asks a number of questions for each step in the process: (1) How could this process step fail? (2) What are potential causes for the failure? (3) What might be the consequences of the failure? (4) How likely is such a scenario? A risk priority number is then assigned to each failure based on the likelihood of occurrence and the severity of the consequences. In this way, the failures can be prioritised in terms of the risk they pose.

FMEA is a useful tool in order to understand key vulnerabilities of care processes, so that these can be addressed and controlled before small errors aggregate and cause larger failures or adverse events and patient harm. FMEA has been used in a number of different care settings including intravenous drug infusion (Apkon et al. 2004), blood transfusion (Burgmeier 2002) and emergency care handover (Sujan et al. 2014a). However, there has also been criticism of the approach in healthcare, suggesting that it was time-consuming (Dean Franklin et al. 2012), demonstrated low reliability when used by different teams (Shebl et al. 2009), and that the focus on single errors might not be adequate to capture the complexity of real failure scenarios in healthcare (Sujan and Felici 2012). It is worth bearing these criticisms in mind, but arguably the benefit of adopting an approach such as FMEA comes from the proactive discussion around potential failure opportunities within a multi-disciplinary team in a systematic and structured fashion. Investing in such activities is a prerequisite for enhancing the reliability of care processes to higher levels, and it is a key component of mindful organising.

Enhancing resilience – Performance variability

Reliability and safety

Improving the reliability of care processes by exerting greater managerial control over processes and behaviours is a useful start. However, in order to achieve higher levels of safety, and to aspire to the performance of ultra-safe industries such as commercial aviation, this is not enough. Reliability is not the same as safety and being more reliable does not necessarily mean being safer. For example, once a patient's waiting time in the emergency department approaches the breach threshold, staff and managers might be tempted to revert to practices and shortcuts aimed at meeting the target (i.e., performing reliably), but which might pose additional risks to the patient's safety.

The reason why reliable performance does not by itself guarantee safe performance lies with the complexity of many modern systems, including healthcare (Hollnagel 2014b); see Chapter 3 for an introduction to systems theory, with application to healthcare. Healthcare systems are characterised by changing demands and finite resources giving rise to competing organisational priorities, such as the management of patient flows and time-related performance targets (Sujan et al. 2015a). Healthcare systems might be regarded more appropriately as systems of systems (Harvey and Stanton 2014) or complex adaptive systems (Braithwaite et al. 2013). For such systems, it is not possible to specify upfront every possible scenario and required form of response and behaviour.

In order to succeed, such systems require a certain degree of flexibility and adaptability to deal with changes, surprises and the unknown. As a result, HROs need to do the opposite of the previous step – they need to be able to relinquish excessive managerial control and embrace performance variability. Successful organisations operating in complex environments are those that are able to manage effectively this trade-off between managerial control through simplification, standardisation and anticipation of known risks on the one hand, and flexibility and adaptability through performance variability, on the other hand (Sujan et al. 2015b).

Resilience

Recent literature in the area of resilient healthcare provides many examples that the way everyday clinical work is unfolding – referred to as work-as-done (WAD) – is necessarily different from what those who design and manage healthcare systems assume – referred to as work-as-imagined (WAI) (Hollnagel et al. 2013; Wears et al. 2015; Braithwaite et al. 2016a). This is because healthcare professionals are able to make dynamic trade-offs and to adjust their performance in order to meet changing demands and deal with disturbances and surprises (Hollnagel 2014a,b; Sujan et al. 2015a,b; Fairbanks et al. 2014). Empirical studies of everyday clinical work provide a diverse range of examples of such performance adjustments in practice (Debono and Braithwaite 2015; Sujan et al. 2015c; Braithwaite et al. 2016b).

One specific example comes from the study of handover in emergency care, where clinicians need to make many different trade-offs (Sujan et al. 2014a, 2015a). For example, when ambulances are queuing at the emergency department, ambulance crews might handover their patient to another crew waiting in line in order to save time. The second crew will then be less familiar with the patient when they eventually handover the patient to the emergency department staff. Ambulance crews in this instance are trading the risk of not meeting clinical need in the community due to queuing with the risk of having a poor quality handover from a crew who are not familiar with the patient. The empirical work demonstrated that clinicians resolve such tensions dynamically and sometimes in violation of the formal time-related performance target, based on the specifics of the situation and on their sense of 'being worried' about the patient in their care (Sujan et al. 2015b, 2015c).

Such necessary performance adjustments contribute to organisational resilience (Fairbanks et al. 2014) by adding the adaptive capacity that is required to operate successfully in complex environments. From a WAI perspective, on the other hand, performance variability is often regarded as detrimental deviations or violations (Hollnagel 2015). The challenge for organisations is to manage this seeming contradiction mindfully.

Organisational learning – Sustaining progress

HROs are learning organisations

The principles of mindful organising suggest that, first and foremost, HROs are learning organisations (Hopkins 2007). Encouraging active reporting by staff, demonstrating a commitment to listen and providing the necessary resource and infrastructure for acting on concerns underpin mindful organising.

Organisational learning can be characterised as a continuous cycle of action and reflection (Carroll and Edmondson 2002). Organisations might be more successful at learning from past experience if they create and foster the capacity for deep reflection on whole system dynamics, which can lead to fundamental change (Argyris and Schön 1996). On the other hand, insistence on past traditions, and quick fixes to existing strategies and procedures might inhibit more powerful forms of organisational learning. Organisations have a range of learning processes at their disposal, which might be internal (e.g., audits and adverse event reviews) as well as external (e.g., feedback from the regulator) (Popper and Lipshitz 1998).

Many organisations are relying on incident reporting systems as a key process for reporting and organisational learning (Drupsteen and Guldenmund 2014; Le Coze 2013; Lukic et al. 2010). Ideally, effective learning from incidents triggers improvements in practice that enhance safety and productivity (Lukic et al. 2012). The analysis of incidents seeks to reveal contributory factors and underlying causes (Drupsteen and Guldenmund 2014), which can then be addressed in order to reduce the likelihood of incidents recurring. Learning from past experiences does not have to be limited to the consideration of incidents, but can also include monitoring and analysis of leading indicators, or even weak signals (Drupsteen and Wybo 2015). However, there is increasing evidence in the literature that suggests that effective learning from past experiences in order to improve safety performance remains challenging even in traditional safety-critical industries (Le Coze 2013; Lukic et al. 2012; Drupsteen and Hasle 2014).

The challenges of organisational learning in healthcare

Following the public inquiry into the failings at Mid Staffordshire NHS Foundation Trust in England, the subsequent Berwick report generated lessons and suggestions for change for the UK government and the National Health Service (NHS) in England (National Advisory Group on the Safety of Patients in England 2013). The report recommends that the NHS should aim to become a system devoted to continuous learning and improvement of patient care. This is clearly a fundamental requirement for any healthcare organisation aspiring to improve the safety of care to higher levels.

Incident reporting as an instrument for organisational learning was introduced into the NHS about 13 years ago, following a publication by the Department of Health (2000). This report recommended the development of a reporting system based on the model of incident reporting used in commercial aviation. Incident reporting is well established in the NHS, and it is regarded as a key instrument for improving patient safety and the quality of services (Barach and Small 2000; Anderson et al. 2013).

In one respect, incident reporting in the NHS has been very successful. There are a staggering number of incidents reported every year. However, despite the large number of potential learning opportunities, questions have been raised about the effectiveness of incident reporting systems to contribute to improvements in patient safety (Sujan and Furniss 2015; Pasquini et al. 2011; Braithwaite et al. 2010; Macrae 2015; Vincent 2004). There are now many studies that document barriers to effective incident reporting in healthcare. Such barriers include, for example, fear of blame and repercussions, poor usability of incident reporting systems, perceptions among doctors that incident reporting is a nursing process, lack of feedback to staff who report incidents and lack of visible improvements to the local work environment as a result of reported incidents (Braithwaite et al. 2010; Macrae 2015; Benn et al. 2009; Lawton and Parker 2002; Sujan 2012; Sujan et al. 2011). Among management staff in particular, there continues to be widespread misperception that incident reporting systems might be useful for monitoring incident frequencies, despite evidence that suggests that incident reporting data are poor indicators of actual incident frequencies (Westbrook et al. 2015). It has been suggested that the focus of learning from incidents in healthcare has been too much on collecting and categorising data (Macrae 2015; Anderson and Kodate 2015), whereas successful learning from experience should inherently be a social and participative process (Lukic et al. 2012; Macrae 2015).

Learning from the ordinary

How can healthcare organisations enhance their ability to learn from past experience in order to set them on the path towards becoming an HRO, given the obstacles and practical difficulties with learning from incidents outlined earlier? One way might be to shift the focus from formal learning about extraordinary failures and incidents towards more decentralised, local forms of learning about everyday clinical work (Sujan 2015).

An example of such a local form of learning is the Proactive Risk Monitoring in Healthcare (PRIMO) approach. This approach to organisational learning was developed in order to elicit a rich contextual picture of the local work environment, to move away from negative and threatening notions of errors and mistakes, and to encourage active participation and ownership with clear feedback for local work practices (Sujan 2012; Sujan et al. 2011). The distinguishing feature of the PRIMO approach is that it focuses on learning from the ordinary, in this case the various hassles that practitioners experience in their everyday clinical work. See Box 7.1 for a detailed account of the PRIMO approach.

Box 7.1 Case study: Proactive risk monitoring in healthcare

Incident reporting is well established in the NHS, and the English National Health Service National Reporting and Learning System (NRLS) was established in 2003. The main focus has been on reporting harms after they have happened which are then used to predict future risks. However, high-reliability principles suggest that risk can be managed more effectively through a social and participative approach that anticipates and monitors the conditions that create risk.

The PRIMO project drew on principles of high reliability from the oil and gas industries to proactively identify processes that might contribute to risk without depending on incident or accident reporting (Hudson et al. 1994). PRIMO uses staff narratives about day-to-day working and 'hassles' in their workplace to identify the priority areas for monitoring in the local context. These are thematically analysed and a set of Basic Problem factors are selected for regular monitoring. These Basic Problem factors are monitored monthly through a staff survey leading to a risk profile of the workplace.

Areas that can be quickly resolved are prioritised and improved, giving staff confidence that the system does lead to tangible improvements and action plans for more complex problems are devised and their success evaluated by the monthly monitoring survey.

Staff narratives are collected every 3 months to elicit new Basic Problems to be included in the monthly monitoring. This iterative process meant that the risk profile was updated in real time and staff felt ownership for the process as well as seeing the consequences, all leading to an improvement in the safety culture.

One of the test sites for PRIMO was a radiology department of a district general hospital (DGH) with approximately 240 beds. The radiology department consists of the main x-ray department and a number of specialist modalities such as computed tomography (CT), magnetic resonance imaging (MRI) and nuclear medicine. The whole department employs approximately 90 staff. Some of these are employed part time. The roles within the department range from clerical, radiographic assistant, assistant practitioners, radiographers, specialist radiographers, advanced practitioners and consultants.

(Continued)

Box 7.1 Case study: Proactive risk monitoring in healthcare (*Continued*)

Over the course of the 12-month implementation period, 70 narratives were collected. The analysis identified the following problem areas:

High-level factor	Example from narrative
Communication and Information	'Work closely with A&E – must be some better way for organising the return of patients to the A&E department. Quite often we are just looked at when we return patients on trolleys, as no one seems to know which cubicle the patient is going back to'.
Equipment and Computers	'This week I have worked in the general x-ray department performing many A&E examinations. I have noticed the standard of A&E trolleys are of poor quality, and the faults make it difficult for radiographers to perform the examinations. One of the handles on one trolley is broken so there is nothing to hold onto whilst pushing the trolley. The bucky trays are quite stiff on some trolleys; you could trap your fingers'.
Staffing	'Staff are constantly taken out of the main department to cover other modalities. General rooms can be understaffed and patients put at risk due to constant demands'.
Demand, Management and Workload	'Patient booked for a long list of examinations as a General practitioner (GP) referral on a Saturday morning, when there are only 2 members of staff on duty for emergencies and limited GP examinations. This should have been booked for a week day'.
Work Environment	'Rooms are left untidy, meaning the next person taking over has to tidy the room before they can begin an examination'.
Procedures	'Better access to protocols for imaging, more up-to-date; very difficult for new staff as protocols at other departments may have been very different'.
Teamwork and Attitudes	'Sometimes I can feel bullied by people because they are aggressive and demoralised'.
Training	'There are times when process of booking in on reception goes wrong meaning some patients may get missed. Process may need reviewing or ensuring adequate training for staff'.

The staff surveys identified information and communication, staffing levels and the physical work environment as the key concerns. The local improvement team agreed on a number of improvement activities based on this staff feedback.

One of the improvement activities concerned inadequate external communication with the emergency department for patients requiring referral. This relates to patients with a recent history of trauma, who had been referred by their general practitioner (GP), and who may require referral to the ED following the imaging results. There was no communication and decision pathway for these patients and delays in referring patients may occur. This can contribute to poor patient experience, and it requires additional time of staff in the radiology department, which in turn can have knock-on effects on other patients.

Prompted by the data generated through the PRIMO process, a working group with the ED was set up, and a referral pathway and corresponding documentation were developed. The referral pathway has been implemented; staff feedback suggests that the

(*Continued*)

> **Box 7.1 Case study: Proactive risk monitoring in healthcare (*Continued*)**
>
> new pathway is easy to use; there have been no issues raised from the ED, suggesting that the pathway works for all stakeholders.
>
> The PRIMO tool demonstrates the high-reliability principle of continuous organisation learning can be applied to healthcare setting with ease and to good effect.
>
> Source: Adapted from Sujan, M. and Cooke, M., *Proactive Risk Monitoring in Healthcare (PRIMO): Prerequisites for Deployment in Diverse Settings and the Impact on Safety Culture*, Health Foundation, London, 2014b.

Hassle in this instance can be defined loosely as anything that causes people problems during their daily work. Examples of hassle include, for instance, unavailable equipment such as drip stands on a ward or supporting equipment for undertaking radiographic procedures. There are a number of important benefits of learning from everyday hassle. Among these, the most important benefit is arguably that the focus on hassle supports building an understanding of the system dynamics, that is, of the way performance adjustments are made, and the way work ordinarily unfolds. Reports of hassle typically contain not only descriptions of how the hassle manifested itself, but also how people coped – how they adapted their behaviour in order to continue to provide safe and good quality care (Sujan et al. 2015b). Examples of typical adaptations made by healthcare professionals include the sharing of information and personal negotiation to create a shared awareness, prioritisation of goals and of activities, and offering and seeking help.

Other local and informal processes that organisations might consider supporting include regular staff meetings aimed at identifying ways to improve the delivery of care, informal discussions between staff and their managers, and discussions among peers and informal lunchtime improvement groups. Such processes are perceived as locally owned, and they might be better suited to provide shared awareness, to make staff feel that they are being listened to and that they can make a contribution to improving patient safety, and for generating ownership for improvement interventions (Sujan 2015).

Research suggests that where organisational effort is invested to support and include such processes, these can have a positive effect on staff engagement in reporting and learning activities (Sujan 2012) and on patient safety (Goldenhar et al. 2013). Utilising a range of processes that draw upon and strengthen different aspects of an organisation's culture might enable healthcare organisations to deliver more sustainable improvements in patient safety (Singer and Vogus 2013).

Conclusion

Some industries and organisations have a remarkable safety track record despite operating complex technology in hazardous environments. The study of how such organisations manage safe operations over long periods of time has given rise to the theory of HROs and a corresponding model of mindful organising. A mindful organisation is characterised by a strong commitment to reliability, resilience and organisational learning.

The path towards becoming an HRO is challenging, and the journey requires vision, leadership and an organisational culture of safety and improvement. Experiences from industry suggest that even in ultra-safe organisations this remains a challenge and a daily struggle.

Healthcare systems, such as the NHS in England, have made progress with patient safety, but much more needs to be done to reassure patients that the care they receive is safe. The reliability of processes can be improved using a number of established process improvement and risk management tools. The importance of resilience and the positive contribution of performance variability are only now starting to become recognised in healthcare. This might lead to greater authority and responsibility being given to frontline staff for improving services. Similarly, organisational learning has been recognised as a priority, but it has been managed centrally through formal structures, such as incident reporting systems, and with limited success. Healthcare organisations need to explore how they can provide support to less formal, locally owned mechanisms for organisational learning.

Organisations do not become HROs overnight. Improvement can start locally, in any area of an organisation. Key to this is always individuals, local champions, with a strong desire to improve the safety and quality of care delivered to patients.

References

Anderson, J.E. and Kodate, N. (2015) Learning from patient safety incidents in incident review meetings: Organisational factors and indicators of analytic process effectiveness. *Safety Science* 80: 105–114.

Anderson, J.E., Kodate, N., Walters, R., and Dodds, A. (2013) Can incident reporting improve safety? Healthcare practitioners' views of the effectiveness of incident reporting. *International Journal for Quality in Health Care: Journal of the International Society for Quality in Health Care / ISQua* 25: 141–150.

Apkon, M., Leonard, J., Probst, L., DeLizio, L., and Vitale, R. (2004) Design of a safer approach to intravenous drug infusions: Failure mode effects analysis. *Quality and Safety in Health Care* 13: 265–271.

Argyris, C. and Schön, D.A. (1996) *Organisational Learning II: Theory, Method and Practice*. Reading, MA: Addison-Wesley.

Baker, G.R., Norton, P.G., Flintoft, V., Blais, R., Brown, A., Cox, J. et al. (2004) The Canadian Adverse Events Study: The incidence of adverse events among hospital patients in Canada. *Canadian Medical Association Journal* 170:1678–1686.

Barach, P. and Small, S.D. (2000) Reporting and preventing medical mishaps: Lessons from non-medical near miss reporting systems. *BMJ (Clinical research ed)* 320: 759–763.

Benn, J., Koutantji, M., Wallace, L., Spurgeon, P., Rejman, M., Healey, A. (2009) Feedback from incident reporting: Information and action to improve patient safety. *Quality and Safety in Health Care* 8: 11–21.

Braithwaite, J., Clay-Williams, R., Hunte, G., and Wears, R. (2016b) Understanding resilient clinical practices in emergency department ecosystems. In: Braithwaite J., Wears R., Hollnagel E., editors. *Resilient Health Care III: Reconciling Work-as-Imagined and Work-as-Done*. Farnham: Ashgate, pp. 115–132.

Braithwaite, J., Clay-Williams, R., Nugus, P., and Plumb, J. (2013) Healthcare as a complex adaptive system. In: Hollnagel E., Braithwaite J., Wears R., editors. *Resilient Health Care*. Farnham: Ashgate, pp. 57–73.

Braithwaite, J., Wears, R., and Hollnagel, E. (2016a) *Reslient Health Care III: Reconciling Work-as-Imagined with Work-as-Done*. Farnham: Ashgate.

Braithwaite, J., Westbrook, M.T., Travaglia, J.F., and Hughes, C. (2010) Cultural and associated enablers of, and barriers to, adverse incident reporting. *Quality and Safety in Health Care* 19: 229–233.

Brennan, T.A., Leape, L.L., Laird, N.M., Hebert, L., Localio, A.R., Lawthers, A.G. (1991) Incidence of adverse events and negligence in hospitalized patients. *New England Journal of Medicine* 324: 370–376.

Burgmeier, J. (2002) Failure mode and effect analysis: An application in reducing risk in blood transfusion. *Joint Commission Journal on Quality Improvement* 28: 331–339.

Carroll, J.S. and Edmondson, A.C. (2002) Leading organisational learning in health care. *Quality and Safety in Health Care* 11: 51–56.

Carroll, J. and Rudolph, J. (2006) Design of high reliability organizations in health care. *Quality and Safety in Health Care* 5: i4–i9.

Clay-Williams, R. and Colligan, L. (2015) Back to basics: Checklists in aviation and healthcare. *BMJ Quality and Safety* 24: 428–431.

Davis, P., Lay-Yee, R., Briant, R., Ali, W., Scott, A., and Schug, S. (2002) Adverse events in New Zealand public hospitals I: Occurrence and impact. *New Zealand Medical Journal* 115: U271.

de Vries, E.N., Ramrattan, M.A., Smorenburg, S.M., Gouma, D.J., and Boermeester, M.A. (2008) The incidence and nature of in-hospital adverse events: A systematic review. *Quality and Safety in Health Care* 17: 216–223.

Dean Franklin, B., Shebl, N.A., and Barber, N. (2012) Failure mode and effects analysis: Too little for too much? *BMJ Quality and Safety* 21: 607–611.

Debono, D. and Braithwaite, J. (2015) Workarounds in nursing practice in acute care: A case of a health care arms race? In: Wears R., Hollnagel E., Braithwaite J., editors. *The Resilience of Everyday Clinical Work*. Farnham: Ashgate.

Department of Health. (2000) *An Organisation with a Memory*. London: The Stationery Office.

DeRosier, J., Stalhandske, E., Bagian, J.P., and Nudell, T. (2002) Using health care failure mode and effect analysis: The VA National Center for Patient Safety's prospective risk analysis system. *Joint Commission Journal on Quality Improvement*. 28: 209, 248–267.

Drupsteen, L. and Guldenmund, F.W. (2014) What is learning? A review of the safety literature to define learning from incidents, accidents and disasters. *Journal of Contingencies and Crisis Management* 22: 81–96.

Drupsteen, L. and Hasle, P. (2014) Why do organizations not learn from incidents? Bottlenecks, causes and conditions for a failure to effectively learn. *Accident Analysis and Prevention* 72: 351–358.

Drupsteen, L. and Wybo, J.-L. (2015) Assessing propensity to learn from safety-related events. *Safety Science* 71: 28–38.

Fairbanks, R.J., Wears, R.L., Woods, D.D., Hollnagel, E., Plsek, P., and Cook, R.I. (2014) Resilience and resilience engineering in health care. *Joint Commission Journal on Quality and Patient Safety/Joint Commission Resources* 40: 376–383.

Francis, R. *(2013) Report of the Mid Staffordshire NHS Foundation Trust Public Inquiry*. Available from: http://www.midstaffspublicinquiry.com/report (accessed on 12 January 2017).

Goldenhar, L.M., Brady, P.W., Sutcliffe, K.M., and Muething, S.E. (2013) Huddling for high reliability and situation awareness. *BMJ Quality and Safety* 22: 899–906.

Harvey, C. and Stanton, N.A. (2014) Safety in system-of-systems: Ten key challenges. *Safety Science* 70: 358–366.

Haynes, A.B., Weiser, T.G., Berry, W.R., Lipsitz, S.R., Breizat, A.-HS., Dellinger, E.P. et al. (2009) A surgical safety checklist to reduce morbidity and mortality in a global population. *New England Journal of Medicine* 360: 491–499.

Hollnagel, E. (2014a) Is safety a subject for science? *Safety Science* 67: 21–24.

Hollnagel, E. (2014b) *Safety-I and Safety-II*. Farnham: Ashgate.

Hollnagel, E. (2015) Why is work-as-imagined different from work-as-done? In: Wears R., Hollnagel E., Braithwaite J., editors. *The Resilience of Everyday Clinical Work*. Farnham: Ashgate.

Hollnagel, E., Braithwaite, J., and Wears, R.L. (2013) *Reslient Health Care*. Farnham: Ashgate.

Hopkins, A. (2007) *The Problem of Defining High Reliability Organisations*. Working Paper 51, National Research Center for Occupational Safety and Health Regulation. Canberra: Australian National University.

Hopkins, A. (2014) Issues in safety science. *Safety Science* 67: 6–14.

Hudson, P., Reason, J., Wagenaar, W., Bentley, O., Promrose, M., and Visser, J. (1994) Proactive a tripod-delta: Proactive approach to enhanced safety. *Journal of Petroleum Technology* 40: 58–62.

Jones, D.T. and Mitchell, A. (2006) *Lean Thinking for the NHS*. National Health Service (NHS) Report, London.

Kapur, N., Parand, A., Soukup, T., Reader, T., and Sevdalis, N. (2016) Aviation and healthcare: A comparative review with implications for patient safety. *JRSM Open* 7: 2054270415616548.

Kohn, L.T., Corrigan, J.M., and Donaldson, M.S. (2000) *To Err Is Human: Building a Safer Health System*. Washington: The National Academies Press.

La Porte, T.R. (1996) High reliability organizations: Unlikely, demanding and at risk. *Journal of Contingencies and Crisis Management* 4: 60–71.

La Porte, T.R. and Consolini, P. (1998) Theoretical and operational challenges of 'high-reliability organizations': Air-traffic control and aircraft carriers. *International Journal of Public Administration* 21: 847–852.

Lawton, R. and Parker, D. (2002) Barriers to incident reporting in a healthcare system. *Quality and Safety in Health Care* 11: 15–18.

Le Coze, J.C. (2013) What have we learned about learning from accidents? Post-disasters reflections. *Safety Science* 51: 441–453.

Leonard, M., Frankel, A., and Simmonds, T. (2004) *Achieving Safe and Reliable Healthcare: Strategies and Solutions*. Chicago: Health Administration Press.

Lewis, P.J., Dornan, T., Taylor, D., Tully, M.P., Wass, V., and Ashcroft, D.M. (2009) Prevalence, incidence and nature of prescribing errors in hospital inpatients: A systematic review. *Drug Safety: An International Journal of Medical Toxicology and Drug Experience* 32: 379–389.

Lukic, D., Littlejohn, A., and Margaryan, A. (2012) A framework for learning from incidents in the workplace. *Safety Science* 50: 950–957.

Lukic, D., Margaryan, A., and Littlejohn, A. (2010) How organisations learn from safety incidents: A multifaceted problem. *Journal of Workplace Learning* 22: 428–450.

Macrae, C. (2015) The problem with incident reporting. *BMJ Quality and Safety* 25(2): 71–75.

McGlynn, E.A., Asch, S.M., Adams, J., Keesey, J., Hicks, J., DeCristofaro, A. et al. (2003) The quality of health care delivered to adults in the United States. *New England Journal of Medicine* 348: 2635–2645.

National Advisory Group on the Safety of Patients in England (2013) *A Promise to Learn – A Commitment to Act*. London: Department of Health.

Ovretveit, J. (2009) *Does Improving Quality Save Money?* London: Health Foundation.

Pasquini, A., Pozzi, S., Save, L., and Sujan, M.A. (2011) Requisites for successful incident reporting in resilient organisations. In: Hollnagel E., Paries J., Woods D., Wreathall J., editors. *Resilience Engineering in Practice: A Guidebook*. Farnham: Ashgate, pp. 237–254.

Popper, M. and Lipshitz, R. (1998) Organizational learning mechanisms a structural and cultural approach to organizational learning. *Journal of Applied Behavioral Science* 34:161–179.

Pronovost, P.J., Berenholtz, S.M., Goeschel, C.A., Needham, D.M., Sexton, J.B., Thompson, D.A. et al. (2006) Creating high reliability in health care organizations. *Health Services Research* 41: 1599–1617.

Roberts, K.H. (1990) Some characteristics of one type of high reliability organization. *Organization Science* 1: 160–176.

Roberts, K.H. (1993) Cultural characteristics of reliability enhancing organizations. *Journal of Managerial Issues* 5(2):165–181.

Shebl, N.A., Franklin, B.D., and Barber, N. (2009) Is failure mode and effect analysis reliable? *Journal of Patient Safety* 5(2): 86–94.

Singer, S.J. and Vogus, T.J. (2013) Reducing hospital errors: Interventions that build safety culture. *Annual Review of Public Health* 34: 376–396.

Sujan, M.A. (2012) A novel tool for organisational learning and its impact on safety culture in a hospital dispensary. *Reliability Engineering and System Safety* 101: 21–34.

Sujan, M. (2015) An organisation without a memory: A qualitative study of hospital staff perceptions on reporting and organisational learning for patient safety. *Reliability Engineering and System Safety* 144: 45–52.

Sujan, M.A., Chessum, P., Rudd, M., Fitton, L., Inada-Kim, M., Cooke, M.W. et al. (2015a) Managing competing organizational priorities in clinical handover across organizational boundaries. *Journal of Health Services Research and Policy* 20: 17–25.

Sujan, M. and Cooke, M. (2014b) *Proactive Risk Monitoring in Healthcare (PRIMO): Prerequisites for Deployment in Diverse Settings and the Impact on Safety Culture*. London: Health Foundation.

Sujan, M.A. and Felici, M. (2012) Combining failure mode and functional resonance analyses in healthcare settings. *Computer Safety, Reliability, and Security* 7612: 364–375.

Sujan, M. and Furniss, D. (2015) Organisational reporting and learning systems: Innovating inside and outside of the box. *Clinical Risk* 21: 7–12.

Sujan, M.A., Habli, I., Kelly, T.P., Pozzi, S., and Johnson, C.W. (2016a) Should healthcare providers do safety cases? Lessons from a cross-industry review of safety case practices. *Safety Science*. 84:181–189.

Sujan, M.A., Ingram, C., McConkey, T., Cross, S., and Cooke, M.W. (2011) Hassle in the dispensary: Pilot study of a proactive risk monitoring tool for organisational learning based on narratives and staff perceptions. *BMJ Quality and Safety* 20: 549–556.

Sujan, M., Pozzi, S., and Valbonesi, C. (2016b) Reporting and learning: From extraordinary to ordinary. In: Braithwaite J., Wears R., Hollnagel E., editors. *Resilient Health Care III: Reconciling Work-as-Imagined with Work-as-Done*. Farnham: Ashgate.

Sujan, M., Spurgeon, P., and Cooke, M. (2015b) The role of dynamic trade-offs in creating safety – A qualitative study of handover across care boundaries in emergency care. *Reliability Engineering and System Safety* 141: 54–62.

Sujan, M., Spurgeon, P., and Cooke, M. (2015c) Translating tensions into safe practices through dynamic trade-offs: The secret second handover. In: Wears R., Hollnagel E., Braithwaite J., editors. *The Resilience of Everday Clinical Work*. Farnham: Asghate, pp. 11–22.

Sujan, M., Spurgeon, P., Inada-kim, M., Rudd, M., Fitton, L., Horniblow, S. et al. (2014a) Clinical handover within the emergency care pathway and the potential risks of clinical handover failure (ECHO): Primary research. *Health Service Delivery Research* 2.

Sutcliffe, K.M., Paine, L., and Pronovost, P.J. (2016) Re-examining high reliability: Actively organising for safety. *BMJ Quality and Safety*.

Thomas, E.J., Studdert, D.M., Burstin, H.R., Orav, E.J., Zeena, T., Williams, E.J. et al. (2000) Incidence and types of adverse events and negligent care in Utah and Colorado. *Medical Care* 38: 261–271.

Vincent, C.A. (2004) Analysis of clinical incidents: A window on the system not a search for root causes. *Quality and Safety in Health Care* 13: 242–243.

Vincent, C., Barber, N., Franklin, B.D., and Burnett, S. (2009) *The Contribution of Pharmacy to Making Britain a Safer Place to Take Medicines*. London: Royal Pharmaceutical Society of Great Britain.

Vincent, C., Neale, G., and Woloshynowych, M. (2001) Adverse events in British hospitals: Preliminary retrospective record review. *BMJ (Clinical Research Ed.)*. 22:517–519.

Wears, R., Hollnagel, E., and Braithwaite, J. (2015) *The Resilience of Everyday Clinical Work*. Farnham: Ashgate.

Weick, K. and Sutcliffe, K. (2007) *Managing the Unexpected: Resilient Performance in an Age of Uncertainty*. San Francisco, CA: Jossey Bass.

Westbrook, J.I., Li, L., Lehnbom, E.C., Baysari, M.T., Braithwaite, J., Burke, R. et al. (2015) What are incident reports telling us? A comparative study at two Australian hospitals of medication errors identified at audit, detected by staff and reported to an incident system. *International Journal for Quality in Health Care: Journal of the International Society for Quality in Health Care / ISQua* 27(1): 1–9.

Womack, J.P., Jones, D.T., and Roos, D. (1990) *The Machine That Changed the World*. New York, NY: Free Press.

8 Implementing Healthcare Improvement

Susan Went

Introduction

Knowing what best practice is and being able to put it in place are two different activities. This chapter explores the practical implementation at a local level.

There are many different triggers to improvement. One example is a child learning to ride a bicycle. This usually starts through watching others, often siblings and friends. Observing can be a powerful motivator and may well trigger the initial desire to learn, to be part of the peer group and join in. But desire alone is not enough and listening to parents and friends helps understanding and appreciating what to do and what not to do, how to get the seat in the correct position and why a helmet is important. The learning may also be underpinned by parental incentives and rules: 'If you learn to ride properly we will buy you a bike', 'if you don't do it safely you will not be allowed to do it'. Practical experience of the real thing, the trial and error of falling off and experiencing bruised shins and grazed knees together with the exhilaration of success will all add to the learning. This learning may continue as the child seeks higher levels of achievement through more formal teaching and undertaking a recognised cycling proficiency test, watching elite road and track racing such as the Tour de France and the Olympics. Ultimately, this might lead to the experience of cycling in different terrains or taking up cycling as a competitive sport.

As discussed in Chapter 3, healthcare is both complex and complicated meaning that the situations and circumstances within healthcare vary too much for a standardised 'drag and drop' approach to implementing improvement. The metaphor of learning to ride a bicycle and becoming increasingly proficient is a powerful illustration of the application and implementation of improvement science in practice. As with all applied learning, it takes the learning from the classroom into the real world, ensuring that students 'learn by doing'. It does not abandon theoretical knowledge rather it moves students from passive to active learning and from abstract to concrete knowing.

Objectives

The chapter's objectives are to:

- Consider how the development of a local theory of change model for a specific improvement can help with putting improvement into practice
- Explore how quality improvement can be scaled up across multiple sites
- Understand the factors involved in sustaining improvement over time

Improvement in practice

There is growing interest in many countries of what constitutes quality and how to create, high-performing healthcare systems in practice. A 2-year study by Baker (2008) in three countries identified nine key attributes common to healthcare systems that successfully implement quality improvement:

- Outstanding leadership
- Quality and system design defined as a core business strategy
- Investment in building capacity and capability for improvement
- Integration of services across levels of care, sites and disciplines
- Harnessing of information technology and meaningful measurements
- Clear focus on putting patients and clients first
- Engaged workforce (including physicians)
- Strategic alignment of aims, measures and activities
- Alignment of incentives and accountability

Staines (2007) proposed that there are a number of discrete phases to achieving this state that are undertaken sequentially. First, an infrastructure is created, including ensuring the capability of staff to undertake improvement activities. Next, care processes are reviewed and redesigned and once these have been embedded and sustained, improvements in outcomes start to be demonstrated. Both Baker and Staines implied that without investment in building a critical mass of improvement capability and capacity, the likelihood of successful quality improvement projects leading to improved patient outcomes is greatly reduced.

Creating this capacity includes strategic planning to provide the golden thread that makes quality improvement more than a series of isolated projects. Baker (2008) was able to demonstrate how high-performing healthcare systems clearly link each improvement initiative and project to the organisation's core strategy and integrate capability for improvement into their operational delivery system or infrastructure.

Change theory

A wide variety of initiatives and approaches have been used to try and address the recognised quality challenges in healthcare worldwide. Many of these methods have drawn on improvement approaches, which originated outside healthcare, particularly organisational approaches used with the manufacturing, aviation and nuclear industries; these are discussed more fully in Chapter 1.

All improvement theories share a common theme around the need for change. Change theory has its roots in a number of disciplines, including organisational sciences, psychology and sociology, but one of the most well-known and influential is Lewin's three-step model.

Kurt Lewin has had significant impact on the understanding of group dynamics and social psychology. His work included theories on social change (Lewin 1947) including his description of change as primarily a three-step process, which recognised that planned change involves the analysis and rebalancing of the competing driving forces pulling individuals in the desired direction and the restraining forces pushing people in the opposite direction. Lewin's theory marked a shift from technical to behavioural models, focusing on the motivation for human behaviours. It asserts that change takes place when the combined strength of force in one direction is greater than the combined strength of the opposing forces. This may take place spontaneously but can also be planned and managed.

The first stage of Lewin's planned change model is to 'unfreeze' the current position or the status quo. Lewin considers the status quo represents the balance between the existing driving and restraining forces. It is a state of equilibrium and change will not occur unless or until one of three things happens: either the change agent increases the driving forces, decreases the restraining forces or a combination of the two. The role of the change agent is therefore to disrupt the equilibrium. Techniques which may help with unfreezing include:

- Showcasing examples of how things have been done differently together with the benefits gained
- Identifying local champions who may persuade peers around the art of the possible and to try something different. Motivating the individuals and teams affected by including them in problem-solving and the design of solutions
- Removing some of the restraining forces which are creating the barriers to change

Once the status quo has been destabilised, the conditions are ready for stage two when 'change' or movement towards the desired goal takes place. This involves the creation of new drivers through new thoughts, ideas and behaviours allowing individuals and groups to be liberated from the status quo. This may be achieved through:

- Peer-to-peer discussions, listening to stories from colleagues, leaders and patients (Denning et al. 2007) and influential high-profile leaders in the relevant clinical field
- Presenting data to stimulate reflection and discussion
- Using creative thinking techniques such as brainstorming and provocation, for example, the Six Thinking Hats (De Bono 1989), which is a tool for getting groups to consider issues from different positions or 'hats'; for example, the white hat is about information, whereas the red hat is about feelings

The second phase of the model needs to be carefully monitored. Having unfrozen the status quo, there is potential for a range of new practices to be adopted and quality improvers cannot assume that their preferred option will be the automatic choice. The movement towards the new goal is often an iterative process and can take a number of rounds and it is therefore best not to rush to the third stage of refreezing until the change phase has been fully exhausted and optimum processes for the specific setting have been identified.

Once the best practice has been developed and has demonstrated the desired effect, the third stage is to 'refreeze' or cement a new status quo. Refreezing needs to take place to ensure that the change becomes stable, embedded and is sustained and there is no reversion to previous practices that might reverse the improvement. Refreezing may be facilitated by

- Agreeing and codifying new standard operating procedures, policies and procedures
- Creating incentives for working with the new process and/or consequences for failing to do so
- Celebrating advocates for the new way of working and the outcomes obtained

It is important to note that whilst mandates and policies are a key part of the improvers' arsenal, they are most effective when used to refreeze and can act as a restraining force if used too early at unfreeze or change stages. Time spent engaging and informing those affected by the change, including staff and senior sponsors, will help to increase understanding of the driving and restraining forces, the impact of the current process and will help to gain support for the proposed changes. This engagement should also include patients and carers and the wider community. Engaging and involving patients and the public in quality improvement are discussed in Chapter 4.

Box 8.1 presents a hypothetical case study, based on real-life experiences, which demonstrates how 'Sarah-Jane', a therapy manager used Lewin's three-step model to bring about change in a community hospital. The case study refers to driver diagrams, illustrated in Figure 8.1 and explained in more detail in the section 'Driver diagrams'.

Box 8.1 Case study of using Lewin's three-step model to bring about change in a community hospital

Sarah-Jane started her job as therapy manager at St Elsewhere 6 months ago. The hospital was part of an organisation providing community and primary care services. Most of the services managed by Sarah-Jane were working well but there was concern about the flow of patients in the physiotherapy outpatient service. The physical environment for the service was inadequate and there was a constant battle to manage the number of referrals meaning that the waiting list was long and complaints were increasing.

This situation had been developing over several years, so much so that some of the team considered it normal to have patients waiting up to 6 months for treatment. However, Paula, the orthopaedic physiotherapist practitioner, together with some other team members wanted to do things differently but couldn't find a way to resolve the problem. Sarah-Jane was concerned that these experienced staff would leave to work at the larger university hospital if a solution could not be found. Things had to change; this wasn't working for patients, for physiotherapy staff or for the referrers.

Sarah-Jane knew that other outpatient services ran things differently, particularly for musculo-skeletal services (MSK). In these services, the referral and treatment processes enabled staff to assess all new referrals quickly and to allocate patients to the most appropriately skilled practitioners. As a result, these services had seen significant reductions in waiting times, lost appointments and in re-referrals. Both Sarah-Jane and Paula had experience of using quality improvement techniques in the past and agreed that an Improvement project was needed.

Unfreezing

Sarah-Jane set time aside to talk with Paula. She wanted to understand the problem from Paula's perspective and to work together to develop a better process. Paula told Sarah-Jane about a conversation with a young patient in pain and she described how two of the orthopaedic consultant referrers had telephoned her to complain about the service. Sarah-Jane and Paula talked about the referral process itself, the role of the reception staff and how the work was allocated.

Sarah-Jane and Paula started to look at the volume, source and type of referrals received in the last 12 months and sought help from the information department to predict future patterns. They also reviewed the appointment booking templates to work out how many staff and appointments would be required to clear the current waiting list and still meet new referrals which would come in over the same time period. Sarah-Jane

(Continued)

Box 8.1 Case study of using Lewin's three-step model to bring about change in a community hospital (*Continued*)

agreed to send Paula on an advanced quality improvement skills course in order to be able to teach improvement techniques to the staff who would be involved in the change.

Sarah-Jane met the medical staff who made referrals to the service to assure them that she was determined to change things and to seek their input to making improvements. She invited them to join a project steering group which would bring together the people closest to the problem and with the most to gain from finding a new way of working. Nadia, one of the general practitioners (GPs), was keen to introduce a direct referral to physiotherapy triage. Phil, one of the orthopaedic surgeons, was supportive but another surgeon was cynical having tried to get things changed before but been unsuccessful; however, he nominated one of his team to join the steering group.

The following day, Sarah-Jane telephoned four of the patients who had complained about the service to ask if they would be willing to help with some re-design work and two were keen to participate. The organisation's patient advice and liaison service also promised to help.

Sarah-Jane shared her commitment to making improvements with her team and outlined the key points of the project. It became clear that everyone in the room had heard different things in Sarah-Jane's feedback and their responses were influenced by what they thought the issue was. One was adamant that the number on the waiting list was the main problem whilst others argued that it was about length of wait; Paula was keen to stress the impact on her staff and Sarah-Jane was concerned about the reputation of the department and the profession. Everyone agreed that if they had family members waiting for treatment they would think it a very poor service.

Paula suggested turning the next team meeting into a workshop, to try to get a more cohesive view of the problem and uncover the main areas for change. Although she wasn't intending to use theory in the meeting, she could see the workshop as a way to develop a driver diagram (see Figure 8.1).

The meeting generated lots of debate and discussion, producing a general consensus around a measureable goal which was to reduce the waiting time to a defined maximum number of weeks by a given date. The team agreed that the actual maximum wait time should be set not just by the physiotherapists but also by referrers and importantly by patients. The debate also identified several clinical conditions and types of referrals which should be considered separately, for example urgent referrals and pre/post-surgery referrals.

Armed with the draft driver diagram, data from the information team, the patient story and the complaints log, Sarah-Jane's next stop was the divisional senior management team. She knew this would not be an easy meeting and she wanted to be as prepared as possible. Although she knew the clinical director would be influenced by the complaints and patient story, she needed to be able to give 'hard' facts to the operational and finance team. Demonstrating the level of commitment from colleagues and staff was also important, so she invited Nadia, the GP, to come with her to talk about triage models.

(*Continued*)

Box 8.1 Case study of using Lewin's three-step model to bring about change in a community hospital (*Continued*)

It was a difficult but constructive meeting, as with so much evidence of the need to change, the engagement of patients, staff and colleagues, together with a vision for change and the beginning of a logic model, it was possible to discuss the need for additional short-term funding to reduce the current waiting list and support staff training. Emma, the divisional manager, agreed to join the steering group to help to prepare a robust business case for the management team.

Without extra capacity, all new and existing referrals would have to be channelled through the new pathway and whilst a more efficient pathway may reduce waiting time in itself, the backlog of patients awaiting treatment meant that the goal would not be achieved within the financial year and it would therefore be harder to demonstrate the added value. The management team were excited by the proposal but given the financial position could not approve the full funding requested. They agreed that Sarah-Jane could have two not three temporary staff, however Emma allocated some project manager time to prepare the project plan and work along side Sarah-Jane.

Change

Having gained the support and funding, Sarah-Jane set about refining the change process. She tested the draft driver diagram with the information staff and reception colleagues to check that data requirements, referral and scheduling issues had all been properly identified. She checked with transport and portering services to check for any unintended consequences. The steering group reviewed the driver diagram and the project plan to check that all key components had been captured, before signing them off.

Sarah-Jane and the patient volunteers spent time with the senior therapy team to identify the optimal new pathway and wait times. Sarah-Jane then repeated the exercise with the referrer partners. These meetings resulted in a detailed process map for the new pathway, with proposed start dates and a clear list of the changes which were to be tested. The discussions also made it very clear that introducing the pathway was not the goal; the pathway and other changes were the means to delivering improved outcomes and more timely care.

Sarah-Jane and Phil asked the therapy manager from Phil's previous hospital to speak to the steering group and to the physiotherapy team about his experience. Sarah-Jane asked the physiotherapy professional body for practice exemplar sites and she arranged 2-week secondments for four of the orthopaedic therapy specialists so that they could gain experience of working in a different way before making the local change.

Paula, Nadia and Phil, wrote short pieces for the hospital and GP practice newsletters. The driver diagram and two patient stories were used to help illustrate both the need for and the feasibility of the change.

It was then that Sarah-Jane realised that, although they had planned to start the project implementation during the peak holiday period, having two not three additional

(Continued)

Box 8.1 Case study of using Lewin's three-step model to bring about change in a community hospital (*Continued*)

staff meant that the reduction of the waiting list would not be complete before most staff were back at work; they had forgotten to rework the assumptions and factor in the limited space in the department. She and Paula went back to the staff to outline a proposal to extend the normal working day and to offer weekend appointments to clear the list; this did not go down well.

Sarah-Jane knew she needed help and although she felt embarrassed about underestimating the space requirements, she phoned Emma (the divisional manager) to seek advice. Emma knew that extended hours was an important strategic aim for the trust. She agreed to support Sarah-Jane with human resources input and to ask the chief executive and medical director to discuss concerns with the therapy staff. Staff were impressed that they came and that both acknowledged the clinical leadership role that therapists were playing.

Over the next few days, Sarah-Jane and Paula negotiated the introduction of Saturday clinics and an extension to the working day as a 6-month pilot. There was now sufficient space for staff to see the patients.

Fourteen weeks later, with great excitement, the team started to introduce the new pathway. Each change was monitored for its impact on the waiting times and treatment outcomes. As a result of the time they had spent planning and seeking expert advice, there were few problems. Sarah-Jane and Paula took every opportunity to report on the progress and achievements, posting run charts on the department walls so that staff and patients could see the reduction in wait time. Team confidence grew as all the metrics started to move in the right direction.

Refreezing

The patient and clinical teams, who co-designed the new pathway, were asked to review the new processes and the outcomes with the aim of making any further refinements. Once the review work was complete, and the steering group were content, the referral, treatment and reporting processes were consolidated within the hospital, community and GP information technology systems. The administrative and reception staff drew up standard operating procedures so that all members of the team would have access to written guidance of the new pathway and associated processes.

As the change became established, Sarah-Jane and the members of the steering group started to write up the project and their results in preparation for poster presentations for national events and to submission to professional journals.

Paula and her team continued to post run charts in the department and write for the newsletters. Regular in-house quality improvement clinics were run so that all members of therapy staff could learn about techniques and have the confidence to use them.

By now, Sarah-Jane, Paula and the senior therapists had very strong relationships with the MSK teams in the exemplar sites and they started a staff rotation scheme,

(Continued)

Box 8.1 Case study of using Lewin's three-step model to bring about change in a community hospital (*Continued*)

giving junior therapists at St Elsewhere professional development experience of working in a very busy university hospital site and conversely, offering university hospital staff experience of an integrated community and primary care service.

NB: This is a hypothetical case study, based on the real-life experiences of two NHS therapy managers.

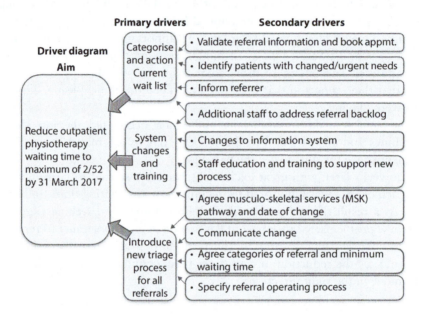

Figure 8.1 Driver diagram.

Local change models

Grand theories of change such as Lewin's provide insights into the principles of how change happens, to determine what works and for whom. The theory needs to be translated from the general to the particular through the development of a local change model. Weiss (1995) suggested that change can only be fully understood if the particular, local, change model is explicitly described and articulated through a program theory (this is discussed in more detail in Chapter 10). This approach has become known popularly as a 'theory of change model'. Articulating a theory of change for an individual improvement project challenges leaders to be specific about the assumptions and logic of their approaches and to clearly articulate the steps they believe will deliver the improvement.

A theory of change model is a description of how the move from the current state to the desired future state will be achieved and as such may be described as a road map. It describes each of the individual interventions, how they will contribute to the desired outcome and why they will work in that particular context. A theory of change model therefore includes a mix of what, how and why.

A local change model is distinct from a traditional action plan, which starts with the current state and moves forwards through actions which determine the outcome. Instead a local change model works backwards from the aim and desired end point by describing the intermediate outcomes which must be in place to deliver the goal. The result is a set of related steps laid out in a series of logical relationships.

In order to articulate a theory of change, it is important to have an appreciation of the system the improvement practitioner is endeavouring to change (reflecting Deming's Profound Knowledge as discussed in Chapter 1). Appreciation of the system will help to ensure full consideration of all the processes which must change to deliver a different outcome and an understanding of the contextual factors within which that system is operating. System awareness will importantly allow for early identification of the possible unintended consequences of some interventions. Understanding the system is best achieved through developing the local change model in collaboration with key stakeholders, ensuring that their knowledge and experience of the system and their subject matter expertise is fully integrated into the theory of change.

Involving those affected by the change in the design of the local change model will also go a long way to ensure that everyone has the same understanding of the aim, the improvement process and the work involved. A robust change model will provide a framework that allows progress to be monitored and shared with colleagues, helping the spread of improvement by giving other teams a plan of action.

Driver diagrams

Communicating the local change model through a visual presentation is an effective way of engaging all stakeholders. The Institute of Healthcare Improvement uses a template for local change models that they call a driver diagram (Provost and Bennett 2015; Institute for Healthcare Improvement 2016). (See Figures 8.1 and 8.2 for a worked example.)

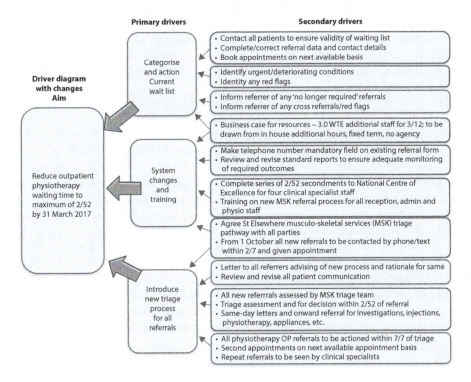

Figure 8.2 Driver diagram after refinements.

The driver diagram has an improvement aim and drivers that are designed to change practice to achieve the aim. Primary drivers are the 'big ticket' items which are believed to have the most significant impact on the aim and these are distinguished from secondary drivers which are associated changes which augment and support the primary drivers. The rationale for distinguishing between primary and secondary drivers comes from the work of the cognitive scientists including Bartunek and Moch (1987) who described three levels of change. First-order changes are those in which a change returns a system to its normal level of performance: there is no permanent change to the aim or outcome. A second-order change is one where change alters the way that the system works to the extent that a new aim or desired outcome is achieved and a third-order change is one in which the system has created the capacity to reflect and dynamically adjust in order to create and maintain excellence.

Creating a driver diagram is a deceptively simple task; the end product will be a clear, visual representation of the steps required, but the process of developing the driver diagram can be protracted and is likely to involve several iterations. Figure 8.1 shows the initial driver diagram that shows the aim of the project. This is then taken and discussed with all the stakeholders in the system and becomes increasingly more refined. Figure 8.2 shows the driver diagram after a number of iterations. When preparing a driver diagram, the flow of work is from left to right; starting with the aim, moving to primary drivers and then to the secondary drivers. It is important not to be tempted to start with the ideas for the process of change, which should be the last part of the methodology, but to agree first on the aim and work backwards.

Even if the general goal has already been defined, it will still need to be shared and the rationale for the change discussed and refined in order to gain consensus with all the stakeholders. It is possible that this process will generate challenge to the original assumptions and it will be important to have access to data to evaluate the challenge and to shape and clarify the goal into a clear aim, which is both specific and measureable, for example:

- By (date, month, year) we will reduce the total number of all falls on the inpatient wards by 60%.
- By (date, month, year), 95% of all patients discharged from hospital care will report that their needs were met.
- By (date, month, year) all referrals for a routine X-ray will be actioned and reported on within 24 hours, irrespective of the referral date.
- By (date, month, year) all patients will be sent a text reminder of their GP or Practice Nurse appointment, 1 week before and 1 day before their appointment.

At the point at which the specific aim has been clearly described and agreed, attention can turn to suggestions about the primary areas of change: the categories (or drivers) that need to be considered to achieve the aim. Although each driver diagram will be unique to its setting, most driver diagrams will share some common areas of action, including changes in processes at the point of care delivery, changes to technology or the working environment and changes in communication flow. Once the primary drivers for change have been identified, work can start on the secondary drivers.

Some of the secondary drivers may have been identified at the early stage but they will probably warrant further exploration and analysis. Less obvious secondary drivers might be made visible through process mapping current and proposed new process (see Chapter 6 for more detail on process mapping).

Once the primary and secondary drivers are described, teams can map the changes required against each one. There are no rules for how many primary and secondary drivers are needed in a driver diagram, and the more complex the project, the more likely it is that the number of primary and secondary drivers will increase.

When mapping a healthcare process, it is important to work with service users to map the whole patient pathway from their perspective, to ensure that the whole system has been considered not just one organisation's delivery pathway. It will be important, for example, to examine whether changes at ward level might impact on other services, such as diagnostics, therapies and portering services, whether changes in outpatient departments impact on primary care or transport or whether changes in primary and community care will impact on social care or on emergency care.

Whilst a local change model describes the logic of the planned changes in an accessible way, it does not guarantee that the logic is correct. It is therefore important to test the assumptions in the local change model during the testing phase. This can be achieved through discussion, gathering data on the intermediate outcomes and questioning the strength of the assumptions about each causal relationship; does x *always* result in y and if not, what are the conditions is which it does not? The testing of the assumptions described by a driver diagram may need a number of iterations over time until the local change model is demonstrated to be achieving its aim.

Spreading and scaling up improvement

Improvement projects and initiatives are a catalyst for change with ambitious and aspirational aims that are both rationally and emotionally engaging; however, 'up to 70% of improvement projects never spread' (Eccles et al. 2012). The challenge, according to Berwick (2004), is that 'in healthcare, invention is hard but spread seems even harder' (Berwick 2004, p. 101). Buchanan et al. (2007) define spread as a process through which new working methods developed in one setting are adopted, perhaps with appropriate modifications, in other organisational settings and they contrast this with sustainability which they define as the process in which methods that have previously been adopted and resulted in performance enhancement are maintained for a period appropriate to the particular circumstance.

Spread of innovations has been extensively described by Rogers (1962), who identified a diffusion curve, with people adopting change at different rates from early adopter through to laggards. In his landmark book *Diffusion of Innovations*, Rogers describes diffusion as a form of communication across a social system and therefore focuses on human decision-making.

Rogers differentiates between the conditions for spontaneous and for planned diffusion. Spontaneous diffusion of innovations is more likely to occur in environments where people have free choice. New technologies for personal use such as social media and smartphones have spread rapidly and spontaneously through individual choice. Spontaneous diffusion is less likely to happen and should not be relied upon, in environments based on formal bureaucracies, such as healthcare systems, which have restraining forces and complex networks that mean personal choice is insufficient for change to occur. Improvement practitioners must therefore actively plan and manage the spread of improvement initiatives and not rely on the gains being implemented because they appear to be self-evident.

A spread strategy should include moving from the initial test site to another similar test site. For example, from one surgical ward to another surgical ward, testing in different clinical specialties, for example, orthopaedic wards, testing at night-time instead of day time and testing at weekend instead of weekday. The stronger the evidence base and the broader the testing, easier it will be to make the case for working at scale and for making the improvement part of everyday work.

In addition to the content of the change, improvement practitioners should also be mindful of the context in which they are seeking to make changes (context is discussed in detail in Chapter 2). The speed at which spread occurs is heavily dependent on the factors that influence an individual's decision to adopt an innovation (Rogers 1962).

In his paper 'Slow Ideas', Gawande (2013) compared the trajectories of two clinical improvements from the nineteenth century, changes in anaesthesia and the introduction of antiseptics, which were both ground breaking innovations with the potential to provide significant improvements in healthcare. One quickly gained traction and spread widely within 9 months, whilst the other took 30 years to become fully accepted.

Gawande describes how the first demonstration of ether anaesthesia in the United States was in October 1846, when William Morton demonstrated a new pain killing gas (ether) to Henry Jacob Bigelow and colleagues. By November of that year, Bigelow had published a paper in the Boston Medical and Surgical Journal and by mid-December that same year surgeons in Paris and London were using ether. By February the following year, it was being used in most centres in Europe and by July 1847 it was being used across the globe. Within 7 years, it was common practice in hospitals in the United States and Europe.

In contrast, Joseph Lister began to explore cross infection in 1860 and proposed that the use of carbolic acid would kill germs and reduce wound infection in surgery. His research continued over the next few years and Lister published his results in the Lancet in 1867. Although the results of his work showed the dramatic impact on this major complication of surgery, his colleagues did not adopt the new idea and the new techniques did not spread beyond a few centres. It was another 30 years before aseptic techniques, including the use of sterile swabs, gowns, gloves and handwashing, became accepted and embedded as routine practice. Gawande proposes that there are clear differences between the two innovations that explain the different speed of the spread. He asserts that the ether-based anaesthesia spread quickly because it addressed an immediate and pressing concern, that of the patient's pain during surgery. The use of anaesthesia, while providing obvious benefit to the patient, also directly improved the experience of the surgeon by allowing them to undertake more complex surgery and in a more controlled manner. In contrast, preventing cross infection failed to attract as much interest from surgeons because it addressed a potential problem that happened after the surgery and therefore after the surgeon had completed his intervention. Whilst preventing infection greatly benefitted the patient, the introduction of aseptic techniques made the surgeons' lives more complicated and unpleasant, as carbolic acid burnt their skin.

Spread and sustaining improvement is therefore dependent on demonstrating both impact and return on economic and human resource investment. Gawande's observations reflect Rogers's findings that individuals weigh up the potential costs and benefits before committing to a change. Improvement interventions with an immediate and positive impact on both patients and staff involved in their care, have more traction and are more likely to spread quickly than changes which are designed to prevent future potential harm or failure; these changes which require more considered persuasion. When seeking to spread quality improvements, it is important to demonstrate that the return is worth the investment. Addressing issues of major concern to staff can gain early support for the improvement; this could include addressing issues that cause staff frustration and that eliminate wasted time. Once staff are engaged, this can serve as a platform for addressing the less tangible but equally important improvements that ensure harm is prevented.

A number of spread frameworks are available (Massoud et al. 2006; Scoville et al. 2016; Maher et al. 2007; Jeffcott 2014), all of which emphasise the importance of leadership and clinical engagement to ensure that improvement is not reliant on spontaneous spread alone.

Depending upon the specific improvement intervention, the following levers may form part of a spread strategy:

Awareness raising

- Developing clinical champions and senior leader engagement
- Establishing a community of interest that creates a critical mass of supporters for culture change
- Data to highlight variations and demonstrate improved outcomes
- Patient pull – informed and empowered patients, creating demand for the improvement to be sustained

Incentives and targets

- Flexible funding/commissioning models (e.g., when there is recognition that costs in one part of the health and care system, or one organisation, lead to savings in another)
- Recognition of success such as conference papers and entry for achievement awards

Mandates and regulation

- Formal levers including responsibilities in employment contracts
- Inspection, using both internal and external assessment criteria

Smoking reduction is an example of a public health initiative which utilised all these levers, to spread health promoting behaviours. It has been known since the mid-1950s that smoking is bad for health and a major cause of lung cancer. This knowledge alone, however, had little effect on smoking rates and a planned change campaign was required.

The first stage was a national campaign of information and awareness raising, including striking television and newspaper adverts showing the damage which smoking causes to lungs and life style alongside health warnings on all packets. This was followed by a consistent and increasing taxation policy, which made cigarettes both more expensive and more difficult to purchase. Lastly, there came a change in the law which made smoking in public places illegal and punishable.

One of the most widely used spread techniques is the use of breakthrough collaboratives. The original model was developed by Batalden in 1994 to help teams to close the gap between 'knowing' and 'doing', by providing a short-term, highly structured approach in which teams and organisations learn together and from each other. Collaboratives rely on a combination of six key elements which are described by the Institute for Healthcare Improvement (2003):

1 **Topic selection:** It is important that the topic selected is based on robustly evidenced interventions. The value in using breakthrough collaboratives is in spreading knowledge which is sound but not widely used.
2 **Faculty recruitment:** Any improvement intervention relies on support and advocacy of respected and recognised champions. The breakthrough collaborative faculty perform this role, defining and leading the content for the improvement work. They help to devise the aims, the metrics and the changes which will be applied in participating sites.
3 **Enrolment of participating organisations:** Organisational engagement in the collaborative is optional, but sign up requires commitment to a set of clear expectations and obligations.

4 **Learning sessions:** Face-to-face learning events for all the teams occur throughout the duration of the collaborative. In the original model, it was proposed that there would be three learning events, spread evenly across a typical collaborative duration of 6–15 months. The events would offer opportunities for understanding the proposed changes, learning about Improvement techniques and measurement for improvement. Importantly the learning sessions would be about sharing results of local tests of change, both successes and failures.

5 **Action periods:** The periods between learning events are defined as action periods, time when the local teams take their learning back to their organisation and test the change intervention, collecting time series data to measure the impact of the changes.

6 **The model for improvement:** Collaboratives by their nature imply collective learning and working on a common joint project. In the breakthrough collaborative model, both the content and the methodology are common across the teams and the common methodology is the model for improvement (Langley et al. 1996).

More recently, the Institute of Healthcare Improvement (2003) has refined their Breakthrough Series model to include more focus on pre-project work to better prepare organisations and teams before the first learning event: and to develop stronger engagement of senior leaders in each organisation in order that frontline successes are supported and barriers are quickly addressed.

The collaborative model is increasingly being adapted from the original initial single topic, single sector concept and is being used to underpin many cross sector improvement programmes lasting for longer durations than the original 6–15 months.

The strength of improvement collaboratives appears to lie in the personal contact, peer support and social networks which underpin the methodology; as such there is benefit to the participating teams who gain knowledge and learning (Greenhalgh et al. 2004). Collaboratives can also help to develop connections between patients and healthcare providers, between care providers and to build 'coalitions for change' (Health Foundation 2014, p. 14), however there is mixed evidence about the impact of improvement collaboratives (Health Foundation 2014).

Scaling up improvements

There can be a temptation to celebrate the first signs of success and improvements are sometimes moved from pilot to scale in quick succession on the assumption that successful outcomes in a local site means that the intervention is the cause. Change is complex and multi factorial. Good outcomes can be associated with poor processes and poor outcomes can be associated with good processes. It is important, therefore, to understand not only if an intervention is successful, but to demonstrate how it was successful: whether the success was because of or in spite of the intervention. Evaluation is discussed in more depth in Chapter 10.

Not all projects are immediately scalable, for example the improvement which is based on additional funds which are limited in duration, will need to have reached a level of maturity which makes the improvements viable without the extra funding before it can be fully scaled up.

The Institute for Healthcare Improvement together with Associates for Process Improvement have published a framework for taking interventions to full scale (Barker et al. 2016). The framework is derived from their study of existing scale up approaches and experience of large scale improvement work in Africa. They identify three major considerations: determining if the initiative is scalable in its current form, the sequence of actions required to scale-up an improvement initiative and the actions which will reinforce the scale-up efforts.

A key element in scale up was found to be the identification of the *scalable unit*. The framework seeks to provide a clear sequence to spread activities:

- **Set up:** The initial step is to define the intervention and to determine the ultimate goal: the ambition of full scale. Identifying the first test site is critical together with establishing champions for the change and determining how progress will be monitored and measured.
- **Develop the scalable unit:** This step requires practitioners to identify the smallest unit within the system, which most closely replicates the conditions for full-scale implementation. The scalable unit must capture the impact that is required at scale and therefore should reflect the bounded system; for example, should the scalable unit be the ward, or does the improvement need pharmacy input and the unit should be the hospital?
- **Test of scale-up:** Once the improvement has been tested in one unit, work will move to other associated settings. The test of scale may move from one clinic to other clinics, from weekday care to weekend care, from day time to night-time. Each new environment will provide useful learning about the transferability of the improvement, about the infrastructure, resource requirements and the system capacity required to scale up the work.
- **Go to full scale:** Finally, building on the substantial learning and evidence base accrued in the previous stages, focus shifts from replication and deployment across the remaining sites and *scalable units*. It is suggested that scaling up is conducted in multiples of five from one patient or one ward or one team; to five patients, five wards or five teams; from there to 25 patients, 25 wards or 25 teams.

Sustaining improvement

Buchanan et al. (2007) described sustainability as changes that are 'maintained for a period appropriate to a given context'. This definition of sustainability as being for an appropriate period of time reflects the fact that quality improvement is iterative rather than a permanent 'refreeze'. Sustainability actions therefore need to avoid the potential for closing down further improvement and innovation whilst avoiding unwarranted variance from what has been demonstrated to improve outcomes. In improvement terms, sustainability is about ensuring that the system does not revert to the 'old' processes as soon as the improvement initiative ends.

Sustainability therefore constitutes a third-order change, in which the organisation or unit is constantly mindful of the usefulness of the improvement and alert to changes in the context that might mean the current processes are not the best practice and recognises the need for change.

Dixon-Woods et al. (2012) found that most improvement project evaluations are roughly concurrent with the duration of the initiative and very few evaluations include follow-up studies and therefore the evidence around sustainability is scant. They concluded that improvement measures need to be embedded in wider mechanisms and to achieve this, changes need to be 'locked in' to the organisational infrastructure. They also noted that other types of organisational change can quickly destabilise progress and reverse achievements unless improvements are fully embedded and so ongoing senior executive support may be required to sustain progress in the face of such challenges.

Bate et al. (2008) highlighted the importance of embedding achievements in organisational, operational and performance mechanisms, to become *business as usual*. Attempts to spread and sustain improvements can be challenged once key personnel leave, particularly if the initiative is too strongly linked to one key individual, as many initiatives evaporate if the key leader moves (Mills et al. 2003). Initiatives supported by senior leaders and improvement work undertaken in environments which have a good improvement infrastructure are more likely to be sustained as they are able to easily automate new processes, adapt standard operating procedures and align incentives and/or professional or educational requirements. Scoville et al. (2016) noted the importance of using quality control mechanisms to sustain improvement and embed progress in the everyday standard work practices. As Juran and Godfrey (1999) did before them, they made the distinction between quality control, the evaluation and control of performance during operations and quality assurance, the assessment and evaluation of operations after the event.

Sustaining improvements takes time, with Staines (2007) suggesting that truly embedding system improvement may take up to 10 years. In order to avoid dropping the ball, quality improvers should spend as much time on their sustainability strategy as on their improvement intervention design. This includes identifying who will continue to monitor the outcomes and how to make the new processes embedded in the 'way we do things around here'.

Conclusion

Grand theory is pivotal to understanding how to improve quality, but on its own it is insufficient to create local improvements. Healthcare is complex and each practice environment is a unique microcosm and so standardised interventions are almost doomed to failure, meaning that those who wish to bring about quality improvement need to be able to adapt both theory and the experience of others in order to deliver similar improvements in their own workplace. This starts with understanding their environment and understanding what is the most appropriate unit of change: being neither too large nor too small but simply just right.

This will identify the stakeholders for the improvement and it is important to share assumptions and develop a consensus of what might work and why. This will inevitably take a number of iterations, and tools such as driver diagrams can help to encourage the conversation. Being clear about the improvement journey will allow progress along the way to be monitored to increase the probability to success.

Improvement is ultimately delivered by humans and understanding what influences their behaviours is as important as knowing the science behind the intervention to be implemented. It is also important to avoid mistaking early successes for long-term, third-order change and so building monitoring of the improvement in to day-to-day operational management is pivotal to sustained improvement.

The need for individualised improvement designs means that improvement at scale requires a high level of engagement and skills at the direct care interface and change cannot be planned and delivered by a specialised team. Quality is, after all, everybody's business.

References

Baker, G.R., MacIntosh-Murray, A., Porcellato, C., Dionne, L., Stelmacovich, K. and Born, K. (2008) *High Performing Healthcare Systems: Delivering Quality by Design*. Toronto: Longwoods Publishing Corporation.

Barker, P.M., Reid, A., and Schall, M. (2016) A framework for scaling up health interventions: Lessons from large-scale improvement initiatives in Africa. *Improvement Science* 11: 12.

Bartunek, J.M. and Moch, M.K. (1987) First order, second order and third order change and organizational development interventions: A cognitive approach. *Journal of Applied Behavioural Science* 23(4483): 500.

Bate, P., Mendel, P.J., and Robert, G. (2008) *Organizing for Quality: The Improvement Journeys of Leading Hospitals in Europe and the United States*. Abingdon: Radcliffe Press.

Berwick, D. (2004) *Escape Fire*. San Francisco, CA: John Wiley & Sons.

Buchanan, D., Fitzgerald, L., and Ketley, D. (2007) *The Sustainability and Spread of Organisational Change; Modernising Healthcare*. Abingdon: Routledge.

De Bono, E. (1989) *Six Thinking Hats*. London: Penguin.

Denning, T., Kelly, M., Lindquist, D., Malani, R., Griswold, W.G., and Simon, B. (2007) Lightweight preliminary peer review: Does in-class peer review make sense. *ACM SIGCSE Bulletin* 39(1): 266–270.

Dixon-Woods, M., McNicol, S., and Martin, G. (2012) *Overcoming Challenges to Improving Quality*. London: Health Foundation.

Eccles, R.G., Perkins, K.M., and Serafeim, G. (2012) How to become a sustainable company. *MIT Sloan Management Review* 53(4): 43–50.

Gawande, A. (2013) Slow ideas: Some innovations spread fast. How do we speed the ones that don't? *Annals of Medicine. New Yorker*, July 29 issue.

Greenhalgh, T., Robert, G., Macfarlane, F., Bate, P., and Kyriakidou, O. (2004) Diffusion of innovations in service organizations: Systematic review and recommendations. *Milbank Quarterly* 82(4): 581–629.

Health Foundation (2014) *Perspectives on Context*. Original Research. London: Health Foundation.

Institute of Healthcare Improvement (2003) *The Breakthrough Series: IHI's Collaborative Model for Achieving Breakthrough Improvement*. IHI Innovation Series White Paper. Boston: Institute for Healthcare Improvement.

Institute of Healthcare Improvement (2016) *How Do You Use a Driver Diagram?* Boston: Institute for Healthcare Improvement. Available from: http://www.ihi.org/education/ihiopenschool/resources/Pages/Activities/GoldmannDriver.aspx

Jeffcott, S. (2014) *The Spread and Sustainability of Quality Improvement in Healthcare*. Learning Resource. Edinburgh: Healthcare Improvement Scotland.

Juran, J.M. and Godfrey, A.B. (1999) *Juran's Quality Handbook*, 5th edn. New York, NY: McGraw-Hill.

Langley, G., Nolan, K., Nolan, T., Norman, C., and Provost, L. (1996) *The Improvement Guide*. San Francisco, CA: Jossey Bass.

Lewin, K. (1947) Group decisions and social change. In: Newcomb, T.M., Hartley, E.L., editors. *Readings in Social Psychology*. New York, NY: Henry Holt.

Maher, L., Gustafson, D., and Evans, A. (2007) *NHS Sustainability Model and Guide*. Coventry: NHS Institute of Innovation and Improvement.

Massoud, M., Nielsen, G., Nolan, K., Schall, M.W., and Sevin, C. (2006) *A Framework for Spread: From Local Improvements to System-Wide Change*. IHI Innovation Series White Paper. Cambridge, MA: Institute for Healthcare Improvement.

Mills, PD., Weeks, WB., and Surott-Kimberly, BC. (2003) A multi-hospital safety improvement effort and the dissemination of new knowledge. *Joint Commission Journal on Quality and Safety* 29: 124–133.

Provost, L. and Bennett, B. (2015) *What's Your Theory? Driver Diagram Serves as Tool for Building and Testing Theories for Improvement*. Cambridge: Institute for Healthcare Improvement. Available from: http://www.ihi.org/resources/Pages/Publications/WhatsYourTheoryDriverDiagrams.aspx.

Rogers, E. (1962) *Diffusion of Innovations*. New York, NY: Free Press (accessed on 9 January 2017).

Scoville, R., Little, K., Rakover, J., Luther, K., and Mate K. (2016) *Sustaining Improvement*. IHI White Paper. Cambridge, MA: Institute for Healthcare Improvement.

Staines, A. (2007) *Lessons from Leading System Transformation*. Lyon: Lyon IFROSS Universite Jean-Moulin Lyon.

Weiss, C.H. (1995) Nothing as practical as good theory: Exploring theory-based evaluation for comprehensive community initiatives for children and families. In: Connell, J., Kubisch, A., Schorr, L., Weiss, C., editors. *New Approaches to Evaluating Community Initiatives, Concepts, Methods, and Contexts*. Washington, DC: Aspen Institute.

9   Sharing Healthcare Improvements: Presenting and Communicating Improvement Results

Helen Crisp

Introduction

This chapter focuses on sharing and disseminating improvement work. This is an essential aspect of improvement beyond the actual implementation. However, it is often overlooked, with the combined pressures of delivering healthcare services in challenging contexts, responding to top-down targets for the health service, plus people's interest and enthusiasm for moving on to the next thing:

> Effective communication is critical to successful large-scale change. Yet, in our experience, communications strategies are not formally incorporated into quality improvement (QI) frameworks.
>
> (Cooper et al. 2015)

Sharing results and providing a detailed narrative of your work is very important to enable other improvers to learn from your experience so that successful improvement has a better chance of being replicated. It also facilitates the honest discussion of challenges and approaches that did not work well, avoiding unhelpful duplication of interventions that have not proved successful. Planning for dissemination needs to be included from the outset, with considerations for the time and resources needed. In addition to sharing and disseminating results at the end of the implementation phase, the benefit of communicating the improvement intervention as it is planned and piloted is explored and the ways that this can enhance organisational awareness and 'buy-in' to the work.

The chapter gives suggestions on how to capture the essential information as you go along and the tools and techniques that can support this. It covers the ideal structure for an improvement report, which is the core description of your work and report of the results, on which all other dissemination materials are based. This includes use of reporting guidelines that can help you produce a finished product that is more likely to be accepted for publication. We also consider the many other channels for sharing improvement work beyond the world of peer reviewed journals and the practical ways you can encourage others to build on your work, through training guides or implementation toolkits. Finally, this chapter suggests some ways in which to track and monitor the spread of ideas, so that you can start to gauge the impact of your work.

Objectives

This chapter's objectives are to explain how to:

- Capture the essential information
- Communicate improvement as you do it
- Write up an effective improvement report
- Plan for publication and dissemination
- Consider other approaches to sharing the work: toolkits, training and online learning
- Assess impact of dissemination activities

Capturing the essential information

Information and data capture from the outset

In order to be able to share your experience of improvement work, it is vital that you keep good records of the work, from initial ideas through the planning, piloting and implementation stages, together with robust and relevant data over this period. Once an improvement is successfully made, it soon seems as if 'we always did it like that' and it is hard to remember the stages of implementation and adjustments made along the way. In order to demonstrate that your change has been an improvement, you will need to have robust measures of processes and outcomes, with a clear rationale of how these measures link to the work undertaken and any improved results. Before any change is made, it is essential for baseline measures to be taken, definitely before starting implementation but if possible even before there is a firm plan for implementation. As an intervention is discussed, along with ideas about how to change ways of working, these changes can start to come into place before an official 'start date'. Once implementation is underway, true 'baseline' data can never be recaptured.

Deciding your measures and the data sources

Good quality data are crucial to demonstrate the initial status of the issue which the QI intervention was designed to address, whether a change has happened and to analyse if this has been an improvement. Measures appropriate to the intervention need to be agreed and the data sources, data collection and monitoring systems designed into the intervention from the start. It is extremely hard in practice to manage effectively the data aspects of an improvement project and this is consistently reported as a major barrier. Customised data collections tend to be highly work-intensive and constitute an added burden of work for frontline staff. This can cause resentment of the improvement intervention. On the other hand, relying on routinely collected data can be frustrating, as it may not be possible to retrieve local data submitted to a central collection. Even when the data are available, there may be long time lags or gaps in the data. What was thought to be a 'good enough' measure for the intervention might turn out not to be sensitive enough to measure the changes on the ground. It is rare for the frontline staff working on QI to have in-depth skills to interpret data or access to expertise in data analytics. This can lead improvers to introduce biases or draw incorrect conclusions. If this is not spotted early on, flawed interpretation of data can undermine all subsequent claims to have made an improvement.

Narrative sources of information

The write-up of an improvement intervention should be based on a wide range of narrative sources, including all the key documentation that has been used to design and plan the intervention and support its implementation in practice. This is likely to include the initial proposal, project initiation documentation, logic models and/or driver diagrams setting out how the intervention was intended to effect the required change, the overall project plan and subsequent versions as this has been updated. It will also include notes from project meetings and any updated reports circulated to project participants, the management group or an external funder. In addition, it is very helpful to record the stages of plan-do-study-act (PDSA) cycles and other QI techniques used. From the outset consider how the documentation is helping to build the narrative of the project, capturing changes to the design and methods as you go along. If you leave considerations of writing up until the implementation is complete, it is hard to remember the course of decisions and why changes were made.

Keep a reflective journal

A reflective approach to the research process itself is accepted practice in qualitative research. Keeping a reflective journal throughout the process of planning and implementing an improvement intervention is a way to make your experiences, opinions, thoughts and feelings visible as an acknowledged part of the research process and to enable you to use this in writing up the work.

Why keep a journal?

Reasons for keeping a journal include:

- To keep a detailed history of your improvement intervention
- To track the development of your improvement skills and understanding
- To provide a context for reflecting on improvement and the problems it highlights
- To enable you to have an overview of progress over a period of time
- To provide a reference point for what happened when in the process

The reflective journal may be a helpful way to think through and articulate the theory of change for the intervention: why you are planning certain elements in your intervention and how you expect it to work. You can record how you decided on your methods as being appropriate for the intervention, work through the implications of the chosen approaches and consider in a critically reflective way who will benefit from the improvement. Michelle Ortlipp writes:

> One of the concrete effects of keeping and using a critically reflective research journal, in which I wrote about my emerging understanding of research methodologies and reflected on different views about gathering (or generating) data, was that changes were made to the research design.
>
> (Ortlipp 2008)

What to include in the journal?

The types of information and reflections to include in the journal include:

- The improvement activities on a day to day basis
- Summaries of discussions about the work

- Notes of books and papers that are informing your thinking
- Ideas that you want to follow up
- Notes and diagrams to form the theory of the intervention
- Analysis of issues or problems that are emerging
- Action plans for next stages

It is important to choose a format keeping the journal that is easy, accessible and comfortable for you to use, whether this is in a notebook, on a computer or notes on your smart phone. If it is inconvenient to open the journal to make notes, it will become a chore to record your thoughts and hard to maintain in a practical way. The journal needs to be at hand as thoughts and reflections occur to you. Aim to make an entry every day you work on your project; although the amount you want to record will vary, it is not helpful to try to standardise the journal entries. Rounding this up with weekly or monthly reviews helps maintain momentum and to identify emerging trends.

Communication of the work as it develops

Communication as a key component of improvement work, as it happens, is often overlooked. The focus for communication tends to be at the point of writing up, publication of journal articles and considering the ways in which the results can be disseminated once the intervention has demonstrated the desired improvement. This is very important, but in order to reach the stage where successful work can be reported, ongoing communication can be one of the success factors. Involving people through communication, as the work develops can add to that success. Communication needs to be considered as a two-way process, not restricted to pushing out information about the improvement intervention and your plans, but also using the communication to gather the views of other stakeholders, using these to shape the design and responding to diverse reactions to the work.

Communicate your plans early

There is a temptation to wait until there is a 'finished product' before sharing plans, but by involving people early on in the planning process for your improvement intervention, there is the benefit of testing the ideas across a range of different perspectives. Patients and service users will have their own views about how they would like to see services improve and what would make the most difference from their perspective. Likewise, staff in other parts of the service will have a view and may raise concerns about how your proposals might impact on their work, upstream and downstream in the patient pathway from where the change is proposed. Rather than seeing this as an irritation, early communication gives the opportunity to model the improvement and make adjustments that can overcome potential negative 'knock-on' effects.

Communicate with senior managers and opinion leaders

The importance of support from the chief executive and senior management is emphasised in improvement literature as a key factor for successful implementation (Dixon-Woods et al. 2012). Involving organisational leaders from the outset means that they are more likely to support the work as challenges arise during implementation and at the stage where sustainability requires a transition from 'improvement project' to 'business as usual' for the way the service is organised. Communicating your plans with the leaders and seeking input means that you are better able to position the improvement so that it aligns with organisational and external policy drivers. These are key factors for long-term success (Halladay and Bero 2000).

In addition to the management leadership, there will be key people who are opinion leaders in your organisation and who may be at any level in organisational structures. It is important to identify and work with the people who have this influence and to think about the people they will respect and listen to. In this way, you choose the appropriate change champions to communicate your work to the opinion leaders. For example, it is often useful if a doctor committed to the improvement intervention presents the ideas to other doctors. Likewise, it may be helpful if support staff communicate to their peers. Remember that this communication needs to be a two-way process, providing *and* gathering information. These interactions provide essential opportunities to test how the proposed improvement intervention is perceived by staff groups and to explore ways in which it may challenge existing work practices or be seen to threaten additional work for certain staff. Early communication provides the opportunity to address these issues at the outset.

Use existing networks and communication channels

Healthcare organisations are highly complex with myriad activities and projects at any time, so the attention and 'airspace' available to communicate improvement work is quite limited. It is therefore important to use the existing communication channels, such as regular newsletters, e-mail bulletins and team briefings to share what you are doing. Alongside these 'official' communication channels, there will be many formal and informal professional networks where information spreads through social diffusion: conversations between peers, use of social media to share good practice tips and coffee catch-ups which can all be used to share key points of your improvement work. However, the content and style of information need to suit the communication channel, so don't try to shoehorn project objectives, timescales and data reports into informal/social channels. These are more suited to the interesting nuggets about what is working well, patient feedback and staff reaction to the intervention.

Writing up an effective improvement report

The improvement report is the key text that gives the narrative of your improvement intervention: the issue that it was designed to address, your methods, the measures used, the results and an analysis of the change that was introduced. The fundamental questions that the improvement report should seek to answer are 'Why did you start? What did you do? What did you find? What does it mean?' as set out in *Writing and publishing in medicine* (Huth 1999).

Once a full report is drafted, the information can be edited and repositioned for presentation in a number of different forms, such as journal articles, newsletter items, conference presentations and good practice repositories, with each of these highlighting different aspects of the work appropriate to the different channels and audiences.

Too many improvement interventions are not reported at all or poorly written up, thus militating against their usefulness as sources of information for improvers in healthcare. It can be quite difficult to get improvement reports published in academic journals, as the work does not always meet the requirements for research journals. Alongside this limitation, reports may be incomplete as a source of guidance to carrying out a similar intervention. Reports of improvement interventions may miss key elements which explain what the intervention was, how it was intended to work, or information about the context where the intervention was implemented. All or any of this would help readers to decide if it is an approach that would be likely to work in their healthcare setting.

Ensure that the write-up of the improvement work takes account of a range of views, not just the programme leader. Involve all members of the implementation team in the drafting of the report. Different perspectives will highlight key pieces of information. No one person can know everything that has happened or the genesis of each adaptation that has taken place over time. It is also extremely powerful to include patients'/service users' perspectives. Include a range of views, not just glowing endorsements but experiences that highlight how service users may have been challenged by new approaches, such as changing the way they access a service or new roles of staff.

A very important aspect of writing up QI work is to include a full description of the context where the intervention took place: the type of healthcare setting, the geographical setting (urban, rural, suburban), the organisational context, such as whether it is a new service or a stable institution. It should also include other relevant contextual factors such as the mix of staff involved, whether the work was building on previous developments or a new approach to the issue tackled. In addition to the contextual information, much of the valuable learning in improvement comes from describing the experience of designing and implementing the intervention. This goes against the grain of much scientific writing, especially reporting of clinical trials, which are explicitly designed to rule out context as an element and where the experience of running the trial is not seen as relevant to the clinical results obtained. Therefore, people moving from the world of clinical trials into the world of improvement may need to 'unlearn' the approach they have previously taken to writing up research work.

Using the Standards for QI Reporting Excellence guidelines

In order to combat these issues, the Standards for Quality Improvement Reporting Excellence (SQUIRE) guidelines were developed in 2008 and an updated version issued in 2015 to increase the completeness, precision and accuracy of published reports of systematic efforts to improve the quality, value and safety of healthcare (Davies et al. 2015). The guidelines aim to help improvers produce more comprehensive and consistent reports of their work. It is hoped this will lead to greater breadth and frequency of published reports, thus becoming a useful source of transparent, rigorous accounts of improvement interventions developed and implemented in healthcare.

When writing an improvement report following the SQUIRE guidelines, you will need to consider:

Title: To convey that this is an improvement intervention and the area of healthcare where it was applied. In terms of people searching for work in your field, the inclusion of key information in the title makes it much easier to identify the work through any kind of online search.

Abstract: A brief overview of the work that includes information on the background, the issue addressed, the methods used, your results and conclusions.

Introduction: To include a description of the problem your intervention tackled, a summary of previous interventions and research in this area and the rationale for the way in which you designed and implemented your improvement intervention.

Methods: Include information on the context in which the intervention was implemented. Provide a description of the core components of the intervention and who was involved in implementation and sufficient detail of what you did so that others could reproduce it. Set out the measures that you used to study the processes and outcomes of the intervention and the ways in which completeness and accuracy of the data was assessed. A section on analysis needs to set out the qualitative and quantitative methods used to draw inferences from the data.

Results: Include the data from process and outcome measures and any modifications made in response to the data during implementation. Provide a clear explanation of the association between the components of the intervention and the outcomes observed. For example, in an intervention concerned with hand hygiene, it is important to be explicit about the links from provision of education to an observed change in the rate of hand washing. Report any contextual elements that interacted with the intervention. Also consider unintended consequences, unexpected benefits, problems, failures and any information on the cost of the intervention and how this compares to the cost of usual care.

Discussion: Summarise your key findings and the implications for your intervention and its effectiveness.

The SQUIRE guidelines are free to download from http://www.squire-statement.org/.

Please refer to the online version, not just the summary of items above. The full version includes detailed notes on how to use the guidelines and examples from published articles to illustrate how the guidance has been applied in practice.

Don't wait until you come to the point of writing up your improvement project to download and study the guidelines. In the field evaluation of the SQUIRE guidelines, many authors found the guidelines a valuable aid to planning the improvement intervention (Davies et al. 2015). The guidelines also provide a useful checklist to ensure that essential information is collected as implementation goes along.

Unlike some other publication guidelines, including Consolidated standards of reporting trials CONSORT (randomised trials), STROBE (observational studies) and PRISMA (systematic reviews), which focus on a particular study methodology, SQUIRE 2.0 is designed to apply across the many approaches used for systematically improving the quality, safety and value of healthcare. Methods range from iterative changes using PDSA cycles in single settings to retrospective analyses of large-scale programmes, to multisite randomised trials (Ogrinc et al. 2015).

The guidelines are a useful tool and prompt but are not intended to be slavishly followed, as this may result in an overlong document and one in which it is hard to pick out the significant pieces of information. When reviewing your work against the guidelines carefully consider the relevance of each SQUIRE item in relation to the improvement intervention. Then consider what it adds to the clarity or rigour of your write up and whether it is necessary to include the item in your report.

A feature of the SQUIRE approach is to get improvement practitioners to consider how they have studied their improvement, as well as how they went about doing the actual improvement work. These are two distinct and equally important activities. When 'doing' improvement work, the motivation is to produce a better service so that patient experience or safety is enhanced, clinical care is better or resources used more efficiently. The aim of studying improvement is to ascertain the transferable knowledge from the local improvement and how this could be applied to improve services more widely. Studying the intervention should allow us not only to know 'does it work?' (Which is sufficient to validate the local improvement) but also to understand the mechanism of how the intervention works, which is essential for any transfer to take place.

SQUIRE 2.0 asks authors to be as transparent, complete and as accurate as possible about reporting 'doing' and 'studying' improvement work, as both aspects are key to scholarly reporting. The 'summary' and 'interpretation' items in the discussion encourage authors to explain potential mechanisms by which the intervention(s) resulted (or failed to result) in change, thereby developing explanatory theories that can be subsequently tested (Ogrinc et al. 2015).

Developing a publication and dissemination plan

Many people working in the field of healthcare improvement are rather shy about promoting their work and being seen to 'blow their own trumpet'. Alternatively, they may see this not as their job but something that other people should be doing. It may not come naturally, but we need to get over this. If we're not thinking out how best to communicate and disseminate ideas about improvement, we're really only doing half the job. As stated at the beginning of this chapter, dissemination planning needs to be considered at the outset of planning your improvement work, not left to the end. The plan needs to consider the audiences you want to communicate with, how best to reach them and therefore the resources of time and money required. The time needed, and particularly whose time, is a crucial question. Clinical leads of successful improvement work often feel overwhelmed by the demands placed on them for dissemination activities. This is compounded by the fact that it is not seen as a legitimate role for a clinical leader. However, the clinical lead, along with patients and service users who have benefitted from the improvement, are the people who others most want to hear from. They are seen as the most trusted sources of information by people interested in adopting their ideas and implementing a similar improvement. Sharing improvement to facilitate the spread of successful approaches is a crucial professional role for all who work in healthcare.

Sharing your improvement work

The following section draws on resources developed by the Health Foundation, which are available to download from the website: http://www.health.org.uk/publication/using -communications-approaches-spread-improvement.

Once you have taken the plunge and are committed to sharing your improvement work through a dissemination plan, a first step is to think about what is likely to make it interesting to others in the field. In order to be attractive to others, ideas for improvement need to demonstrate:

1   Clear advantage compared with current ways
2   Compatibility with current systems and values
3   Simplicity of change and its implementation
4   Ease of testing before making a full commitment
5   Observability of the change and its impact (Rogers 2003)

The relative ease of communication about your intervention will therefore depend on whether it is a relatively small change within a defined area of current practice or a multi-faceted, complex intervention that represents a significant shift for service delivery. Many of the changes that are inherent in improvement interventions tend to be social and relational in nature, rather than a technical innovation. This makes them harder to communicate effectively through channels focused on bite-sized, inert factoids. The key is to hone down the improvement intervention's key principles and the potential benefits of wider implementation.

Developing a communications strategy

Your communication strategy needs to identify:

Objectives:

•   What you want your communications to achieve
•   Spread of information about what you've achieved
•   Encouragement to others to adopt the intervention

- Discussion amongst similar services about the best ways to improve services – perhaps not to take the approach you did, if it was not successful

Audiences: Who you want to reach

- Healthcare professionals in your field
- Patients and service users
- Commissioners of services
- Policy makers

Key messages: The three or four most important pieces of information about the improvement intervention

- How did patients and service users benefit
- How care was made safer, more efficient or more effective

Communications channels: The appropriate ways to reach your identified audiences with messages that are targeted to them

- Professional networks
- Academic and professional publications
- Mainstream media (TV, radio, publications)
- Social media

Timing:

- Planning which communications channels to prioritise
- Consideration of existing communications opportunities and the schedules of these, for example quarterly newsletters, annual conferences
- The timing of the annual commissioning cycle

See the Health Foundation publication *Using Communications Approaches to Spread Improvement* (Health Foundation 2015) for more details: http://www.health.org.uk /publication/using-communications-approaches-spread-improvement.

Prioritising audiences

Improvers often find it easiest to communicate improvement work to their peers, fellow professionals in the same clinical area and others working in healthcare improvement. Whilst these are an important, already interested and likely sympathetic audience, they may not be the most influential in terms of ensuring sustainability of the improvement or even its spread. Use of a simple prioritisation tool considering different audiences will help to focus communications activity where it may be most successful in achieving the communications objectives (see Figure 9.1).

Once you have identified the different audiences you want to reach and their likely level of interest and influence, in terms of being able to help sustain, grow and spread your improvement intervention, think about the different ways you can reach them and also how much effort to put into reaching the different audience groups, linked to their level of influence (see Table 9.1). It is important to use a diverse range of approaches and media. In particular, think

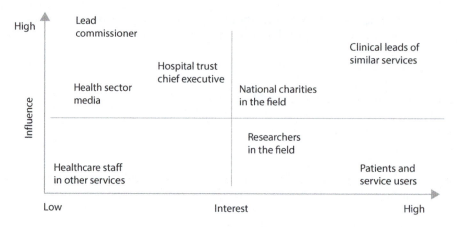

Figure 9.1 Stakeholder mapping for interest and influence.

Table 9.1 Matching communications approaches to category of audience

Audience category	Approach	Communications activity
High interest/High influence	Manage closely	Provide tailored information, hold face-to-face meetings; establish partnerships where appropriate
Low interest/High influence	Keep satisfied	Inform through existing meetings and other channels used by these groups
High interest/Low influence	Keep informed	Provide regular updates through channels used by these groups, consider targeted but infrequent tailored communication
Low interest/Low influence	Monitor	Inform via existing networks and channels such as regular newsletters

Source: Adapted from the Health Foundation, *Using Communications Approaches to Spread Improvement*, Health Foundation, London, 2015.

about where these audiences go for their information, the channels that already exist and use these. For example, use an existing newsletter for patients and service users, rather than produce your own leaflet specifically about the new service or approach. Don't limit your efforts to the written word but think about regular meetings and seminars where you can offer a presentation on the work. Many organisational websites are crying out for more video material, particularly when this includes direct experiences of service users. With today's technology, making a video of reasonable quality is not a major technical challenge. People talking about their experience of the improved service to camera, together with some footage of staff providing the service or of service users doing something they weren't able to do before the improvement, is worth thousands of words of text in a report.

Matching intensity of effort to levels of influence

Another important way to plan your communications and dissemination activities is by thinking about the likelihood of people taking action in response to the information and therefore putting the more intensive effort where this is more likely to engender action. For example, whilst coverage in national media, such as a report in *The Guardian* newspaper, reaches thousands of people and gives a terrific boost to the credibility of local improvement activity, few of the people reading the article are likely to take direct action in response. If *The Guardian* or the BBC contact you, that's great (and is likely to be as a result of some of your targeted dissemination activities) but it's probably not worthwhile investing a lot of time and resources to try to get the attention of national medial channels. On the other hand, if the clinical director of a similar service contacts you, having got the go-ahead in their health system to adopt the intervention (again, probably as a result of targeted information), it is worth putting in time to nurture this interest and respond with quite intensive support. This could involve inviting their staff to observe the work in action, mentoring peers as they plan implementation, sharing your original project plans, procedures, patient information leaflets and so on.

Figure 9.2 shows the different levels of sharing improvement work, linked to the associated methods of communication and dissemination at each level. In the early stages, most effort should be made at the targeted communication level, as this is where the leads will be generated into mainstream media or more intensive work with fellow professionals who are keen to adopt the approach. In addition, use of social media, particularly Twitter, is a good way of sparking interest in your work and linking professional audiences to your targeted communications, such as articles and website content.

As time goes on, and your improvement sustains and has some success in spreading, it is likely that efforts will shift to developing training materials and/or a train-the-trainer approach or developing online learning tools that spread the approach. See the next section on developing training materials and other resources and case study 1 on Practical Obstetric Multi-Professional Training (PROMPT) for an example of this (Box 9.1).

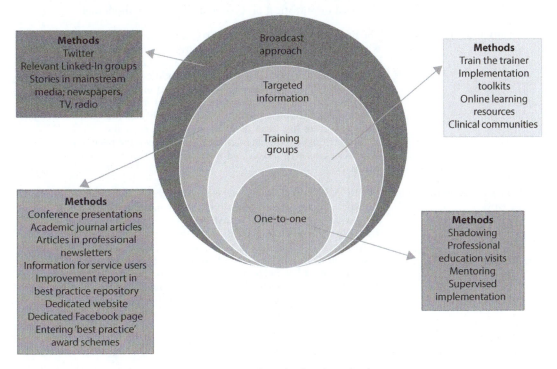

Figure 9.2 Levels of sharing improvement work and related methods.

Box 9.1 Case study: Team training to improve safety in maternity services

Improvement project	*Practical Obstetric Multi-Professional Training (PROMPT)*
Issues tackled and clinical and organisational context	Preventable harm at birth results in serious disability and profound anguish for individuals, families and society. It is also expensive: substandard care and its consequences cost the National Health Service (NHS) in England £3.1 billion in the decade 2000–2010, plus the continuing healthcare costs for these children. The Confidential Enquiry into Maternal & Child Health (CEMACH 1997) reported that there was evidence of substandard care in more than half of all maternal deaths in the United Kingdom, with a lack of multi-professional team working and communication failures identified as contributory factors. In response to these findings, a training package was developed in Bristol (**PROMPT**), designed to improve the outcomes for mothers and their babies during obstetric emergencies. It combines a multi-professional training course with practice-support tools and resources and improvement methodologies in order to bring evidence-based practice to the frontline staff. The programme includes • Teamwork training incorporated in the clinical training. • Quality improvement (QI) methods integrated into the clinical training. • A curated collection of tested local tools, checklists and local standardisation techniques to facilitate best care delivery. • A simple, automated maternity dashboard that provides a monthly display of 12 nationally piloted quality indicators based on statistical process control (SPC) methodologies.
Results and outcomes	The multi-professional training programme implemented at North Bristol NHS trust has been proven to improve knowledge, clinical skills and team working and is associated with direct improvements in perinatal outcome including a 50% reduction in neonatal hypoxic injuries, a 70% reduction in injuries after shoulder dystocia and improvements in performance in Category 1 emergency Caesarean sections. Sustainability of the model and these outcomes has been demonstrated over 12 years. Similar improvements in clinical outcomes have been achieved by other maternity services adopting the PROMPT training approach.
Approach taken to sharing the work	As PROMPT is a training intervention, the obvious way to share the work, and stimulate take up by other maternity units from the outset, was to develop transferable training materials and a 'train-the- trainers' course. PROMPT has very actively used the existing professional networks of clinicians, both midwives and obstetricians. In particular, the Royal College of Obstetricians and Gynaecologists has been a key dissemination partner, selling the PROMPT training manual and being a venue for train-the-trainers courses. The credibility of the training has been enhanced through an active programme of research and publication of academic papers.

(Continued)

Box 9.1 Case study: Team training to improve safety in maternity services (*Continued*)

Improvement project	*Practical Obstetric Multi-Professional Training (PROMPT)*
Examples of communication methods and channels	The clinical results, post-implementation of PROMPT training have been published in high impact journals, including the top clinical research journals in the obstetrics and gynaecology field in addition to journals focussed on medical education, simulation training and quality and safety in healthcare, thus reaching a wide professional audience, not just within the speciality. The training is also promoted through articles in professional newsletters and magazines. There is continued sharing of experience of running the training and the results achieved within PROMPT's own network and also by presentations of different aspects of the work at national and international conferences. Information on PROMPT training and resources is easily accessible through the independent PROMPT Maternity Foundation, with a dedicated website: http://www.promptmaternity.org/.
Response and impact from dissemination activities	PROMPT is widely recognised across the United Kingdom and internationally as a validated team safety training course in obstetrics. Some obstetric units in England have been continuously using and renewing their PROMPT training for over 10 years. It has been mandated for national roll out in Scotland and in Wales and has been taken up by health systems in the United States and Australia. PROMPT has also demonstrated that it can be successfully adapted and implemented in low-resource settings such as Zimbabwe and the Philippines, with demonstrable improvements to safety in maternity services.
	The research work is now investigating the downstream effects of improving clinical outcomes on litigation costs, which are an enormous driver in the developed world.
	The approach to measuring the impact of PROMPT on clinical outcomes has facilitated more sophisticated measurement, leading to the development of an automated system to measure outcomes from routinely collected data at a local level. This Excel-based dashboard is now being piloted and attracting interest from across the globe.
	There is now an undergraduate edition of the PROMPT manual and a new course 'Pre-Hospital PROMPT' for paramedics and community midwives. An app for pre-hospital PROMPT is currently in development.
For more information	http://www.promptmaternity.org/ **Call:** (+44) 0117 323 2322 **E-mail:** info@promptmaternity.org **Postal:** PROMPT Maternity Foundation Department of Women's Health The Chilterns Southmead Hospital Bristol BS10 5NB United Kingdom

Targeted information

As illustrated in Figure 9.2, targeted information is the largest group of dissemination approaches, ranging from academic journals to patient websites. Some are very broad and others relate to a specific audience group and there are multiple channels to reach the same audiences. Communications are likely to have greater impact if a variety of communication methods are used simultaneously and audiences are exposed to the information several times. For example, use Twitter to provide a link to a published article. Don't just tweet it once – use a variety of different messages over a few days. Thereafter look out for people tweeting on similar issues and re-tweet with a link to your article. It may take three or four instances for people to take notice of the information. As long as people don't feel they are being bombarded, the repetition adds to a sense of familiarity and makes the information more acceptable.

Conference presentations

A relatively easy way to get your work in front of fellow professionals is to submit abstracts for poster or oral presentation at relevant conferences. Conference organisers are seeking enough high-quality material to fill the programme, so acceptance rates are in your favour. An oral presentation will tend to have more impact than a poster, but don't pass up the chance of a poster just because you would have preferred the chance to present the work direct to an audience. If your submission is successful, check whether your organisation will support you to attend the conference, through registration fees and time away from work. Usually, only the invited plenary speakers get a free place at the conference. Starting out with general submissions, it is possible to gain recognition to become an invited speaker for a future conference, if your material is original, chimes with the audience and is well presented. In order to increase your chances of a successful submission:

- Highlight where your work links to key themes for the conference (these are often set out in different work streams which makes it easier to see where the work will fit)
- Read the instructions for the particular abstract process and follow this, adapting your material as required by the format – don't copy and paste from a previous abstract submitted elsewhere without considering changes required
- Stick to the word count, which is very limited for most abstract forms: keep background information to a minimum and focus on results and conclusions, whilst including enough information on methods to demonstrate a robust approach
- Ask a trusted colleague not involved in the improvement intervention to review the abstract: is it clear what the intervention is, why it is innovative/original and what are the results?

If your abstract is accepted, make sure you know how long you have to present and be realistic about the amount of information you can convey in the 10, 15 or 20 minutes allocated. You cannot cram everything about a 2-year project into a conference presentation. Decide what will be of most relevance and interest to the audience and focus on this aspect of the work. Many presenters spend too much time going over the background and the methods, running out of time to present their results effectively.

A *word about conference posters*

Most posters displayed at professional conferences are a missed communications opportunity. Don't let yours be one! Remember, a poster is primarily a visual form of communication and time spent considering how design can best highlight the information presented will be well-spent. A poster will only be able to convey a brief snapshot of the improvement work. Consider which aspect to focus on and hone down the information to a few key messages. Again, think about what will be of most interest to the conference audience. Consider the design and how to maximise the visual impact of your work in the way data is presented. Use striking images, which could be illustrations or photographs and ensure that there is space around the text for ease of reading. As few posters adhere to these design principles, producing something outstanding is relatively easy and will attract the attention of people studying the poster boards. Maximise this opportunity by being available near the poster during breaks, so that you can engage interested participants in further discussion about your work.

Conferences are good vehicles for raising awareness about your improvement intervention but in order to turn interest into action, it is a good idea to follow up people who showed interest and share some of your more detailed communication, such as journal articles and links to website content. Encourage them to contact you if they are interested in discussing local implementation or adaptation of your intervention.

Publication in academic journals

There is no doubt that publication of work in peer-reviewed academic journals is seen as prestigious and adds credibility to improvement work. However, this sort of publication is no guarantee of communicating your work to a large audience or stimulating action in response. In your dissemination and publication planning, carefully consider what your aims are in seeking academic publication and make a realistic assessment of the chances of success. In particular, how original is your improvement work and will it meet publication criteria for research if submitted to a research journal?

A good reason for pursuing academic publication is that it will add weight with clinical professionals, especially doctors, if they read about the work in a highly respected journal. Such publication demonstrates that the work has been peer reviewed and judged to have shown appropriate methods and rigour in reporting the results. Academic publication adds to the evidence for the improvement, with questions about 'what's the evidence?' likely to be one of the first challenges raised by clinicians in the face of efforts to spread the intervention more widely. In order to improve the chances of securing publication it is important to:

- Identify the journals most likely to publish your work, either linked to a clinical speciality or because of the methods and approaches used, in which the journal has a regular interest.
- Work through the guidance for authors with a fine toothcomb, to ensure that you have presented the work in the required format and included all requested sections.
- Spend plenty of timing editing and fine-tuning the abstract. This is often neglected, being hurriedly completed at the last minute before submission – but it is the first thing that anyone reads and needs to highlight the key points of interest. Many journal articles are rejected on the strength of the abstract.
- Include enough detail so the reader can understand what you did and how challenges were overcome; without this level of detail the article is not likely to inspire the motivation for follow-up action.
- If you are not used to interpreting and presenting data, get expert help with this aspect. Mistakes in this area will totally undermine claims of successful improvement.
- Identify a suitable peer reviewer familiar with your area of work, if you are asked to suggest peer reviewers.

A complaint of journal editors is that reports of QI work often lack details of the key ingredients of the intervention and the institutional context, so the reader cannot know if the approach is worth pursuing. A typical error is failing to make explicit the links between the problem identified and the specific features of the intervention intended to address the problem. This is the theory for the intervention and enables interpretation of the results as to whether your intervention 'worked' or not. Reports that do not describe any of the barriers of challenges encountered will lack credibility, as readers know that nothing in QI works right away. In the methods section, it is not sufficient to just namecheck 'PDSA cycles' or 'LEAN'. How did you use these methods? What changes were suggested by the 'study' part of the PDSA cycle and how did you plan these and put them into action?

Publication in professional newsletters and magazines

Professional newsletters and magazines may be an easier target for publication, whilst simultaneously having a much broader reach than academic journals. There is a huge range of options here, from national high-profile weeklies like the *Nursing Times*, *Pulse* and the *Health Service Journal*, to very niche magazines and a whole host of e-newsletters and bulletins. Again, you need to target your efforts by considering the audiences you want to reach and their most likely go-to sources for information. It is really worth asking around, particularly of people in other clinical areas and observing what people are reading, or the sources of information they mention in conversation. These publications – whether print or increasingly online – require a different style from an academic article. The focus is on the practicalities and a key interest for readers is the potential to improve services for patients. If you can also suggest how it may reduce staff workload, your intervention is even more likely to be of interest.

As with the selection of academic journals, you need to consider how the target publication appeals to its readers and how your work fits with this. Every article submitted to a different publication needs to be carefully tailored but at the same time will include common elements:

- The issue tackled and why it needed improvement
- The type of healthcare organisation in which the improvement took place, with relevant contextual information
- The design of your improvement intervention, clearly setting out its core components
- How you measured the change you are reporting, but with less technical presentation of data than for an academic journal
- What challenges were overcome along the way
- How patients and service users have benefitted
- Why you would encourage other services to consider this approach

When writing for on-screen media, it is important to use short sentences and paragraphs for ease of reading in that medium. You can also be much more inventive with the use of illustrations, photographs and infographics, which are easier to handle in electronic media.

Award schemes

There are numerous annual award schemes focused on improvement, quality of care, innovation and improving value in healthcare, with some of the best-known national schemes run in association with professional journals: *Nursing Times*, *BMJ* and the *HSJ*. The benefit of such programmes is to boost staff morale and increase the profile and credibility of your work, particularly within your own organisation. If you win or are even shortlisted or commended, this provides a good news story for the organisation. This can then be highlighted to the local media and reported in organisational newsletters, which in turn adds to your credit when you are seeking support for additional resources or to get your improvement commissioned as part of the service offer.

It is not worth investing huge amounts of resource to enter awards. This should not be necessary, as all the key information will already be collated in your improvement report and possibly several existing articles based on the report.

The tips for completing an entry for an award scheme are similar to any other competitive submission:

- Read the categories and entry requirements to see where the work best fits.
- Make a good case for why the work is original and innovative. Awards are often won by a project that stands out because it is doing something really different.
- Clearly explain your improvement approach and methods.
- Highlight your achievements, particularly benefits to patients.
- Even if additional paperwork is allowed, make sure all key information is included in the main submission. Don't make the judges work hard to find this.
- If shortlisted for an interview, think about who will attend. It is powerful to involve patients if possible or a junior member of staff who has made a key contribution, as well as the lead for the work.
- If it is a group interview don't just send one person. This undermines the credibility of the work being a team effort and suggests a lack of interest.

Information targeted to patients and service users

For many improvement interventions, it is just as important to spread the work to patients and to service users as to fellow professionals. This is particularly true where information or awareness-raising is a key component of the intervention. These materials need to be written in nontechnical language, avoiding clinical or health service jargon. A well-written patient information leaflet is often the most widely used communication tool, as the effort to produce a clear, understandable summary of the improvement means that it is suitable to be presented to anyone. For example, patient versions of clinical guidelines are often the ones most used by clinicians, as they present the information in an easy-to-read and quickly accessible format.

Websites and other online platforms

Increasingly, information for patients and service users is going to be most accessible if available online. Many established improvement interventions have developed dedicated websites which include written information on-screen and available as downloadable documents. Online media provide the opportunity for information to be presented in a range of different formats, which may be more appealing, such as video interviews, animations and infographics. A website also enables interactive information-sharing between patients and between health professionals and patients, with the ability to respond to specific queries. Another channel to facilitate easy access for service users is a Facebook page. This has the advantage of being much simpler and less resource-intensive to set up and maintain than a website. The downside is that many NHS organisations are wary of Facebook and similar platforms and how they can be effectively curated, with concerns about the lack of control as to what can be posted.

Online good practice directories

There are many online resource centres, hosted by a variety of different organisations, including National Institute for Health and Care Excellence (NICE) – NHS Evidence, professional associations, professional publications and independent organisations working in particular fields like the major health charities. Some collections assess and select submissions for posting and others are open platforms, some require a subscription or membership before reports can be submitted. In deciding where to submit your quality report, consider your intended audiences and where they are likely to seek best practice ideas and information.

Good practice repositories will usually have their own submission form to complete, to ensure that entries in the collection have some uniformity of presentation and are easy for users to search. As with other formats for sharing information, your core improvement report should include all the necessary information, which can then be extracted and put into the new format. An advantage over journal articles is that good practice collections often facilitate the sharing of additional documentation which can help others adopt the intervention, such as checklists, planning tools and data collection, to name a few.

Sharing information case study

One example of a QI intervention which has successfully shared its ideas through a broad spectrum of targeted information is the PROCEED project in Derbyshire, providing a new style of pre-conception care (PCC) for women with diabetes. Their communications activity has raised awareness of the issues with service users and generated national interest, followed by take-up and adaptation of the approach (see Box 9.2).

Developing training materials and sharing resources

Depending on the complexity and approach of your intervention, sharing the documentation and other resources that support implementation may be an effective way to communicate the work. This approach works best for relatively simple interventions which do not require strict fidelity to the original intervention design and method of implementation in order to work. The type of resources that can be made available include: information sheets for staff and for service users, protocols for the intervention, a checklist, a questionnaire to gain feedback on the intervention, an Excel spreadsheet to report data, a training manual and others. In order to put these materials in context, it is usually helpful to develop a user guide to your intervention. Some good practice resource centres will host this material online together with a report of the improvement intervention, so that other can easily access it.

Developing an implementation toolkit

More complex interventions are likely to require more detailed information and input in order to effectively share the approach. In this instance, a dedicated website for the intervention may be the best way to present and guide access to the material. In this way, all the resources can be provided with contextual information and guidance on their use in practice. The resources are often packed together as a toolkit for implementation. There is also the possibility of including videos that show the intervention in practice and patient stories from people who have benefitted. Don't be put off by the technicalities or potential cost of making a video, as developments in technology mean that this is now cheap and easy. A website also facilitates two-way communication to respond to specific queries and for people to share their experiences of implementation.

Box 9.2 Case study: Preconception care (PCC) for women with diabetes

Improvement project	*Preconception care for diabetes in Derby and Derbyshire (PROCEED)*
Issues tackled and clinical and organisational context	Women with diabetes are two to four times more likely to have a baby with an abnormality and 5 times more likely to experience a stillbirth as women without diabetes. Effective PCC improves outcomes but many women are not able to access this care. The PROCEED project aimed to ensure that women with diabetes received advice and specialist care from pre-conception and through pregnancy to reduce the risk of complications and improve the health of their babies. The project had two components, raising awareness of the need for PCC and delivering user-centred integrated care. For the first, all professionals in contact with women with diabetes were encouraged to use every opportunity to remind women of the need to plan their pregnancy. For the second, timely, accessible care was achieved by changing the setting and staffing of the service from care in a hospital antenatal clinic to offering PCC in group and individual sessions, both in hospital and community settings, with evening appointments available as well as in office hours, together with follow-up by telephone and e-mail. The approach changed the roles of the clinical staff. Specialist nurses and midwives led the sessions, with supervision from a diabetes consultant. Risk profiling enabled the consultant to see women with the most complex care needs.
Results and outcomes	After 12 months, the activity of the service more than doubled, whilst waiting times to access the service went down from 13 to 5 weeks, as the new staffing roles made more efficient use of the limited consultant time. The rate for missed appointments dropped from 18% to 5%. Of women with diabetes who became pregnant, 70% used the service. Many women found it easier and less stressful to attend the sessions in community-based settings than at hospital. The lead roles for specialist nurses and midwives enabled continuity of care. The stillbirth rate for women with diabetes, whilst being cautious about the low numbers involved, has dropped from 5% prior to the introduction of the service to less than 1%. The rate of babies with abnormalities has dropped. In addition to reducing enormous grief and distress for families, the rate of pregnancies resulting in a healthy baby also reduces the costs of ongoing care and treatment. Sustainability of the model and these outcomes has been demonstrated over 4 years. Some economic modelling has been done to estimate the possible savings from reducing congenital abnormalities; potential life-time savings on care and treatment are approximately £18 million.
Approach taken to sharing the work	From early on, the project team, led by Dr Paru King, sought out opportunities to share the work they were doing, as a key objective was to raise awareness of the health risks for women with diabetes and their babies, so that women access care before they get pregnant. The team were keen to share their success with peer healthcare professionals, to encourage adoption of the approach in other localities.

(Continued)

Box 9.2 Case study: Preconception care (PCC) for women with diabetes
(*Continued*)

Improvement project	*Preconception care for diabetes in Derby and Derbyshire (PROCEED)*
Examples of communication methods and channels	The work was promoted to potential service users initially by leaflets, information at structured education sessions and more recently through a dedicated website. The website http://www.derbyproceed.co.uk/ provides information on the PROCEED service for women with diabetes, with pages for healthcare professionals and information for commissioners. Some of the most powerful content is video interviews with women who have used the service and delivered healthy babies. The PROCEED team published their work in a relevant academic journal, *Journal of Diabetes Nursing*, and to reach a wider professional audience in a professional newsletter: *Diabetes Up-date*. Abstracts on the improvement intervention were accepted for a wide range of national and international conferences, focussed specifically on diabetes care and also more broadly on QI in healthcare. Alongside publications and conference presentations, the team entered several awards schemes with some success, winning three awards and getting short-listed for both 'innovation' and 'quality of care'. Success in the award schemes was useful for raising the profile of the work locally and demonstrating that it had been judged as credible.
Response and impact from dissemination activities	PROCEED made the transition from improvement project to commissioned service and whilst this was based on the clinical quality and outcomes of the service, the case for commissioning was undoubtedly supported by the evidence from published academic articles, the video testimony of women who had used the service, the invitations to present the work at major conferences and the credibility of winning national awards. Other diabetes services from around the country have visited Derbyshire to understand how the PROCEED model operates, to take up the idea for local adaptation.
For more information:	http://www.derbyproceed.co.uk/ **Contact:** Dr Paromita (Paru) King, Consultant in Diabetes, Derby Teaching Hospitals NHS Foundation Trust

E-learning approaches

Moving to higher levels of sophistication, there is the potential to develop e-learning materials to share your improvement and to encourage wider implementation. E-learning enables wide accessibility to training and it can be used as a source of income generation. Materials for an e-learning package require a lot of time to develop and will need expert input to translate the concepts from frontline practice into effective online learning modules. Consider from the outset, the plans for where the materials are to be hosted and the dissemination model. Consider whether the module would work as part of a larger course, such as an online Masters' level course in QI. Is it designed as continual professional development for a professional group and could therefore be hosted by a Royal College or professional association.

Once tested, revised and finalised, the online training may not require a high level of input, depending on how it is hosted and promoted. Some approaches include individual tutorial feedback, so be clear from the outset on the delivery model. As a minimum, e-learning providers need to respond to user feedback, amending any sections which do not work well through the online format and ensuring that materials are regularly reviewed and updated as required.

Train the trainer

A more intensive approach is to consider developing training materials to be delivered through a train-the-trainer approach. This gives more control on how the materials are used and tested with trainees so that they understand the concepts and the importance of the core components. It also enables discussion about how far the approach could and should be adapted for local context and to what extent fidelity to the original model is required. An improvement intervention that is either a training-based intervention or requires staff to be trained in particular techniques in order to apply the intervention will lend themselves to a train-the-trainer approach.

Assessing impact of dissemination activities

As set out in the introduction of this chapter, dissemination activities are an essential part of improvement work and should therefore be assessed for impact, just as the impact of the intervention is assessed. By systematically assessing impact across the range of activities, it is possible to know which are most effective for the effort involved and it enables tracking of the spread of ideas and up-take of the work. Having this information available helps to demonstrate the added value to the health system as a whole of the resources used in developing and designing the improvement intervention.

Measuring the impact of dissemination activities is not an exact science and even where it is possible to record numbers of people the information reaches, this does not offer insight as to whether they read it, how they received it or whether they took any action in response. However, it is still worth knowing which website pages were accessed thousands of time and which hundreds of times, what the comparative download figures are for online publications and which conferences have 3,000 participants in the clinical roles that precisely match your target audience.

It is worth keeping records of all the dissemination activities undertaken, categorised as 'conference presentation', 'newsletter article' and 'staff seminar'. Try to get as much information as you can with regard to numbers reached, noting how many people attend a seminar, who they were (midwives, service users, PhD students) and following up with website editors the metrics for numbers of visitors to the web pages, how long the average visit is and the download figures for information materials and other resources. All of this is easily obtainable by anyone with a bit of technical knowledge. When individual professionals contact you for more information, a key measure is to always ask where they heard about the work and add this to your records.

It is acknowledged that what gets measured gets attention, so measuring the impact of your communication and dissemination activities may help to raise the priority of this aspect of improvement work within your organisation.

Conclusion

If we consider that the aim of QI work in healthcare is to improve the overall safety, effectiveness and experience of care received throughout the health service, then the sharing of ideas, knowledge and experience of improvement is important. To present that information in such a way as to encourage the wider application of successful approaches is essential in the face of the major challenges currently facing healthcare, to speed up the adoption of those interventions that really make a difference.

In order to facilitate effective sharing of information, it is essential that the information is captured from the outset and that communication with a wide range of stakeholders is considered an integral part of implementation activities. The information needs to be complete and based on appropriate measures of the change, with attention to data completeness and reliability. Results should be written up in a structured improvement report, which is then the source document for a wide range of other communication and information materials about the intervention.

Be systematic in the way you plan your dissemination of the improvement results and the audiences you are trying to reach. Plan your dissemination strategy from the outset, not as an afterthought once the work is complete and written up. Use a wide range of media to target information to fellow professionals, service users, senior managers and policymakers. The more imaginative you are in identifying communication channels and adapting your presentation and content to the channel, the wider your reach will be.

Always remember, the main purpose of sharing your improvement work is to influence action by others. Your aim is to persuade them to adopt the intervention or to apply the generalisable learning from your work to their own improvement activities. Therefore put the most communication effort into the channels that are most likely to reach those who will take action or have the power to influence wider action.

For top tips see Box 9.3.

Box 9.3 Ten tips for sharing improvement work drawn from the empirical research

1 Get a range of people involved in implementation and dissemination of ideas, including clinical and managerial leaders.
2 View people as active change agents, not passive recipients.
3 Emphasise how initiatives address people's priorities.
4 Target messages differently for different audiences.
5 Provide support and training to help people understand and implement change.
6 Plan dissemination strategies from the outset.
7 Dedicate time for dissemination.
8 Dedicate funds for dissemination.
9 Make use of a wide range of approaches such as social media, opinion leaders and existing professional networks.
10 Evaluate the success of innovations and improvements but also the extent of uptake and dissemination within teams, organisations and more broadly. The things that are measured tend to get more emphasis, so measuring dissemination may help to ensure that it is a priority.

Source: Adapted from de Silva, D., *Evidence Scan: Spreading Improvement Ideas*, Health Foundation, London, 2014.

References

Cooper, A., Gray, J., Willson, A., Lines, C., McCannon, J., and McHardy, K. (2015) Exploring the role of communications in quality improvement: A case study of the 1000 lives campaign in NHS wales. *Journal of Communication in Healthcare* 8(1): 76–84.

Davies, L., Batalden, P., Davidoff, F., Stevens, D., and Ogrinc, G. (2015) The SQUIRE guidelines: An evaluation from the field, 5 years post release. *BMQ Quality and Safety* 24: 769–775.

de Silva, D. (2014) *Evidence Scan: Spreading Improvement Ideas*. London: Health Foundation.

Dixon-Woods, M., McNichol, S., and Martin, G. (2012) *Overcoming Challenges to Improving Quality*. London: Health Foundation.

Halladay, M. and Bero, L. (2000) Getting research into practice: Implementing evidence-based practice in health care. *Public Money Manage* 20(4): 43–50.

Health Foundation (2015) *Using Communications Approaches to Spread Improvement*. London: Health Foundation.

Huth, E. (1999) *Writing and Publishing in Medicine*, 3rd edn. Baltimore, MD: Williams & Wilkins.

Maternal and Child Health Research Consortium (1997) *Confidential Enquiry into Stillbirths and Deaths in Infancy: 4th Annual Report, 1 January–31 December 1995*. London: Maternal and Child Health Research Consortium

Ogrinc, G., Davies, L., Goodman, D., Batalden, P., Davidoff, F., and Stevens, D. (2015) SQUIRE 2.0 (Standards for QUality Improvement Reporting Excellence): revised publication guidelines from a detailed consensus process. *The Journal of Continuing Education in Nursing* 46, (11): 501–507.

Ortlipp, M. (2008) Keeping and using reflective journals in the qualitative research process. *Qualitative Report* 13(4): 695–705.

Rogers, E.M. (2003) *Diffusion of Innovations*. New Yorks: Free Press.

10 Evaluating Healthcare Improvements

Elaine Maxwell

Introduction

With most healthcare organisations now investing in quality improvement, it is important to ask not only did it work but how did it work? Evaluation in healthcare is often considered to be synonymous with audit, but where audit looks at compliance with standards, evaluation looks more widely at the relationship between actions and outcomes and a major task in evaluation is that of differentiating between association and contribution. In the complex arena of healthcare services, it is not sufficient to select a simple pre–post (or before and after) design and to use any differences in data measured to draw conclusions about the impact of the initiative. Unlike the experimental laboratory from which a pre–post design is drawn, in 'real life' situations there are many other potential causes for the observed change. Whilst a single quality improvement intervention can be expected to contribute to some of the change, it is rarely expected to account for all of it. The challenge, then, is to determine both the extent of change and the different factors that might account for it.

Failure to understand the extent and nature of the contribution is part of the reason that repeated studies have shown that quality improvement projects have at best a 30% rate of sustained change (Attaran 2000; Beer and Nohria 2000; Øvretveit 2000; Self and Schraeder 2009; Werkman 2009). Failure to fully evaluate the way in which improvement projects work in specific contexts can lead to a poor understanding of how improvement occurs. This contrasts with clinical care where the understanding of the mechanisms of change is considered axiomatic. Shojania and Grimshaw (2005) noted that whereas no one would prescribe a medicine without a full investigation of the individual patient's problems and a good understanding of how the medicine works, there seem to be a remarkable number of people who are happy to try a quality improvement intervention without an understanding of exactly how it is expected to achieve results. In order for quality improvement to be useful and create lasting change, evaluation must be an integral part of the improvement plan. This chapter concentrates on formal evaluation of programmes, described by Lincoln and Guba (1985, p. 550) as 'disciplined inquiry' and which should be conducted in a manner every bit as rigorous as traditional research.

Objectives

The chapter's objectives are to:

- Explore the nature of quality improvement evaluation
- Consider the choice of evaluation methodologies, their strengths and limitations
- Examine a range of data sources that may contribute to evaluation
- Discuss ways of analysing data collected for evaluation

Approaches to evaluation

Scriven (1967) is credited with introducing the distinction between formative and summative evaluation, formative being a concurrent exercise to aid the process of improvement and summative being an assessment of the impact or effectiveness. Chapter 6 explored how quality improvement is measured during the implementation, and this is often portrayed as the evaluation of the project. Therefore, it might be said that the multiple small tests of theory that are tested through Plan-Do-Study-Act (PDSA) cycles are formative evaluations of specific processes, with the resultant refinement of the hypothesis increasing understanding of the improvement process, rather than simply measuring concordance with the intervention plan. Whilst formative evaluation is undoubtedly important, it rarely makes a strong case for a causal link between the improvement intervention and the change being studied. There is clearly a case then for summative evaluation, including a judgement about the impact that the whole improvement project has had in practice. This chapter focuses on summative evaluation.

Many healthcare professionals will be familiar with Kirkpatrick's (1976) evaluation model. This consists of a four part, linear framework for the evaluation of training programmes and this has been widely used in healthcare professionals' education. The framework follows an idealised chronology of evaluation focus, starting with the students' reactions to the training (what was their perception, did they like it?). This is supplemented by some assessment of their personal learning (what new knowledge was acquired?). Positive perceptions and new knowledge are assumed to lead to a specific behaviour (how did the students' behaviour change?) and it is assumed that this will lead to different results (what was the outcome?). Despite the model's popularity, the first three stages (which are formative evaluations) are conducted far more commonly than the last stage, and this illustrates the challenge of summative evaluation, how can the 'so what?' question be answered? If students enjoy a programme, learn and even change their behaviour, so what if it doesn't change outcomes? Clearly, the mechanism that produces the outcome needs as much understanding as the interventions themselves.

In order to answer the 'so-what question', the evaluation must be situated within the wider system, including socio technical contexts as well as the biomedical factors. The evaluation must be designed around clear questions about the improvement project. There are at least three possible aims of a quality improvement programme evaluation which are relevant for a healthcare professional in practice:

1 Understanding of *the mechanisms* of change (the how) as well as the evidence that the desired outcome (the what) was achieved
2 Identifying whether any observable improvement *is in spite of* a specific quality improvement intervention (i.e., coincidental rather than causal)
3 Understanding whether an improvement is *sustainable* and the conditions in which it might be transferrable

Each of these aims will now be discussed.

Understanding the mechanisms of improvement

The importance of conducting an evaluation of exactly how improvement is achieved in tandem with the measurement of outcomes was well demonstrated at the Hawthorne Works of Western Electric in the 1920s and 1930s (Mayo 1993). The original studies explored whether changes to working conditions would have an effect on worker productivity. Initially increasing the lighting produced improvement but when the lighting was then decreased, productivity increased further. The unexpected finding of the study was that all change increased productivity, at least in the short term. The finding made it apparent that some factor other than the obvious intervention of altering the level of lighting was in play, and it was suggested that productivity increased due to the psychological impact of the attention the workers received from the research team and not because of changes in the experimental variables. More recent analysis has suggested that there were a number of other influences involved, but the fact remains that the initial results appeared to support the original hypothesis that increasing the light increases workers' productivity, and, without further exploration, it would have been assumed that there was a direct cause and effect between increasing workplace lighting and worker productivity. What is clear is that evaluation of any planned change needs a nuanced approach.

A further example of the need to look beyond the immediately visible is the case of the cargo cult phenomenon described by Feynman and Sackett (1985). During the Second World War, large numbers of United States troops arrived on a group of relatively isolated pacific islands. The islanders observed the aircraft descending from the sky and delivering crates full of supplies that American servicemen called 'cargo'. When the war ended, the U.S. troops left and the cargo stopped arriving. The islanders had observed what the troops had been doing and decided to build runways and aeroplanes from local materials such as straw and wood, and they carved wooden radio headsets with bamboo antennae. Once these were in place, they waited for the cargo to arrive. Despite their efforts, no cargo arrived. The islanders had seen empirical evidence that these interventions had worked for the Americans but were unable to replicate it or explain why it had failed for them. The only conclusion could be that something else, less tangible was involved in the process.

It would be easy to dismiss the islanders as naive, but Feynman used this real-life example as a metaphor for people using research findings that rely on the most simple evidence or cherry-pick the most obvious data that supports a desired outcome. There are many examples of quality improvement projects being feted as having improved healthcare based on an incomplete understanding of what actually caused the improvement followed by a disappointing failure to replicate the original results in other settings. A further potential hazard for quality improvers is retro fitting their descriptions of the interventions to accord with the outcomes observed without a substantiated link.

Identifying whether improvement is in spite of the intervention

In many quality improvement projects, there is partial success, and it is necessary to work out which parts of the improvement intervention worked in different contexts and why, rather than throwing the baby out with the bath water. Conversely, without understanding what the causal mechanisms are and whether there was an improvement in some contexts in spite of rather than because of the intervention, it is hard to know which intervention to roll out, and there is a real chance that resources will be wasted by including elements that merely coexist rather than cause the improvement.

Change is the only constant, and there is often an upward secular trend with improvement already happening outside the improvement intervention and being matched by other sites not involved in a particular improvement project. Chen et al. (2016) described how quality problems often surface as a collective concern, and under these circumstances a groundswell of public and professional opinion may be the stimulus for a spontaneous change across a health system. They use the metaphor of a 'rising tide' to describe how an idea starts to gain support and then overtakes planned improvement work and becomes part of the 'zeitgeist' or dominant way of thinking that includes most people's behaviours. This is described by others as a secular trend and if it occurs at the same time as a planned improvement, it can muddy the evaluation leading to improvement in spite of the intervention. Failure to identify a 'secular' change effect needs to be understood to avoid false positive conclusions, and it is inefficient if not unethical to use resources and subject patients to processes that are not adding value. An example of an evaluation demonstrating a concurrent secular trend is Benning et al.'s (2011) evaluation of a quality improvement programme involving four hospitals in the United Kingdom. The results surprised many of the participants by demonstrating that the intervention hospitals, who had received intense training and support, fared no better than control hospitals for reducing rates of patient harm (see Box 10.1).

Box 10.1 The Safer Patients Initiative Programme

The Health Foundation (a British charity) selected National Health Service (NHS) hospitals to participate in a safety improvement project in two phases (Health Foundation 2011). The hospitals were all given mentoring and training by the Institute for Healthcare Improvement (IHI), based on their 'Saving 100,000 lives campaign'. Each hospital had 15–20 'change agents' who were chosen to lead improvement by facilitating the implementation of the programme in their hospital. The change agents received training and support from the IHI.

The programme evaluation was conducted by independent academics who used program theory to design a mixed methods study in which, they tested the intended mechanisms and outcomes of the quality improvement and compared these to 'control' NHS hospitals who did not participate in the scheme. The evaluators used mixed methods including the NHS staff survey to explore perceptions around management support, and the climate of practice as well as examination of patient records, ethnographic observation of practice and secondary analysis of nationally available patient outcome data.

Whilst senior managers at the participating hospitals were greatly enthusiastic about the programme, the evaluators found that staff on the wards generally had only a vague idea of the intervention and few had direct experience of most of its components. There was no significant difference between control hospitals and the Safer Patients Initiative hospitals over time. For some measures, practice was already good at baseline and there was little room for further improvement. There were, however, no consistent trends in either errors or adverse events in medical wards treating patients with acute respiratory disease in the control versus the Safer Patients Initiative hospitals.

The evaluators concluded that the failure to demonstrate a specific advantage to the Safer Patients Initiative might be due to the programme design itself, the implementation of the design or possibly that there were a number of national programmes happening at the same time. They also suggested that the conditions needed to trigger change may have been weak as initiatives sponsored and led by professional bodies, rather than by charities and hospital managers, trigger stronger responses.

Source: Benning et al., *British Medical Journal*, 342, 195, 2011.

Understanding whether improvement is sustainable

The evaluation also might need to consider whether the improvement is sustained and the way in which it develops over time. Greenhalgh et al. (2004) argued that there is a significant gap in the literature in understanding:

> by what processes are particular innovations in health service delivery and organisation implemented and sustained (or not) in particular contexts and settings and can these processes be enhanced? (p. 620)

Van de Ven et al. (1999) described change as a journey rather than a destination and one that is often 'highly unpredictable and uncontrollable' (p. ix) but may be steered in a general direction. Martin (2003) suggested that the complexity of healthcare systems means, change is not a single event but is a continual process. Evaluating the sustainability of an improvement thus needs to take place over time rather than at single points.

As discussed in Chapter 6, many improvement projects are predicated on an iterative cycle of hypothesis testing and small-scale change. Quality improvement is innovative and likely to be very fluid, and it is unlikely that the program theory remains constant throughout. These changes in assumptions and design are hard to ascertain retrospectively and informants may recount their actions through rose-tinted glasses, glossing over some of the key mechanisms involved in the improvement. Improvements may well be achieved through this refinement of the application of interventions rather than the original proposal.

Evaluation methods

The failure to fully understand the reasons for an improvement may be linked to the methods used to conduct the evaluation. Dixon-Woods (2013) observed that the traditional approach to studying causal factors is through using correlational logic; if there are sufficient numbers of cases, the effect of the intervention (the independent variable) on the outcomes (the dependent variables) can be seen. Numerical data is analysed statistically and inferences made. This works well in environments that can be controlled so that the researcher can assume that the intervention is the only variable having an effect and where there are large numbers of cases that smooth out any variations, the gold standard being a randomised controlled trial (RCT). These two requirements, control of environment and large numbers of cases, are rarely in place for quality improvement projects in healthcare and almost certainly will be absent for local improvement projects conducted by individual practitioners and teams.

A further challenge to the use of correlational logic in healthcare quality improvement is that interventions are at least as much, if not more so, social as biomedical. For example, the manufacture of medications results in standardised dosing, but the human element in healthcare means that there can be significant variation in the way the intervention is applied – both variations in the practice of staff and also variation in the way patients choose to apply the advice of clinicians. In addition to variation between individuals, the practice of individuals can vary by time of day, by setting and by workload.

Even if correlation can be demonstrated, Pawson and Tilley (1997) note that this does not necessarily demonstrate causation, nor whether a correlation will be found if the conditions change.

The nature of the issue being improved can also influence the choice of evaluation method. Rittell and Webber (1973) devised a typology of problems ('tame' and 'wicked') to illustrate their differences in order to consider how they might be managed. They suggested that 'tame' problems may be complicated but are well understood and appear to be stable and predictable. A tame problem is one that has occurred frequently and follows the same path each time, and it is therefore reasonable to assume that it can be improved through a standardised, linear sequence of actions which culminate in an outcome in which the problem is fully resolved. Compliance-based approaches to evaluation can work well for tame problems as there is substantial understanding about the mechanism and a low expectation of unexpected variation. An example of this is the IHI's Breakthrough Collaboratives, which were developed to scale up the diffusion and implementation of quality improvement interventions (Kilo 1998). Their programme has been developed around a range of healthcare challenges that were perceived to be well understood and which have been shown to respond to an evidence-based set of actions. Evaluation of such programmes therefore follows a standard design and focuses on compliance with tested actions to achieve predicted outcomes.

On the other hand, Rittel and Webber (1973) suggested that 'wicked' problems are complex as well as complicated. They are by definition ill-defined and less predictable with scant information about the causal factors or of the ways in which the causal factors interact. There is still so much variation in both process and outcome, meaning that the quality improvement intervention is less precise and controlled. They are messy and don't follow a predictable sequence of events and so there is no stable end point which can be identified. Resolving one aspect of a wicked problem often uncovers a previously unseen contributory factor, and therefore the major requirement of the evaluation is to be agile enough to identify unanticipated as well as anticipated causal mechanisms. Evaluation of improvement projects addressing wicked problems are often better served by a theory-driven approach which uses a mixture of data sources and collection methods.

Theory-based evaluation

A theory-based evaluation has well-established questions or a priori constructs derived from the program theory that provide a basis for developing the data collection tools (Eisenhardt 1989), rather than collecting data and hoping that a question will emerge, thus avoiding the potential for 'description without meaning' (Hartley 1994).

Whilst quality improvement has long been linked with theory (it is one of Deming's principles of Profound Knowledge: The theory of knowledge, as discussed in Chapter 1), Stame (2004) noted that policy makers do not adopt programmes solely because of research-based evidence but are influenced by their own bias, assumptions and what the prevailing opinion is for what works. The same may also be said of quality improvement, which can be seen to have developed in a number of different fashions, from audit through Total Quality Improvement to Improvement Science. Stame (2004) noted that there are a number of different approaches to theory-driven evaluation but observes some commonalties between them:

- The evaluation is based on what participants expect to happen.
- Assumptions and values frame the understanding.
- Interventions are studied within their context and rich data is celebrated.
- They use all methods that might be suitable, without privileging any one of them.

In the absence of formal theory, people use practical or pragmatic mind maps when implementing standards and protocols. Practical wisdom is a concept first used by Aristotle to describe the local assumptions developed through both formal knowledge and the practical experience of using it in the real world. Practical wisdom, however, is dependent on individual experiences and may vary between individuals and groups. It therefore needs to be articulated and shared to develop understanding of the drivers for change in a single team or organisation.

Stame asserted that evaluators must try to establish what is inside the 'black box': the space between the actions and the outcome of a programme. The black box can be full of many theories of change that include assumptions and tacit understandings every bit as significant as the research evidence on which the intervention is based and shows the intermediate steps that are triggered by the planned actions, which are rarely articulated but have a profound effect on the outcomes. The black box can be demonstrated through the use of logic models which visually illustrate the logical chain of connections showing what the intervention is intended to accomplish; Box 10.2 explains logic models applied to pressure ulcer prevention.

Weiss (1995) went further and suggested that any social policy evaluation (and quality improvement is largely about social aspects of implementing clinical evidence) must embrace the political environment in which it takes place and she went on to describe the combination of theories into a single 'program theory'. Blamey and Mackenzie (2007) drew a clear distinction between program theory and theory of change, suggesting that program theory makes the assumptions about causal links between actions and outcomes explicit, whereas change theory describes the actions that are anticipated to produce a given outcome but without an explanation as to how they produce the results.

The program theory directs which data are to be collected and therefore should be agreed on before the improvement project starts, because otherwise the workings or mechanism of the intervention may not be captured, leaving the only option: reverting to correlational rather than casual logic. The evaluation is designed to study both whether the intervention worked as the program theory predicted and how the influence of context might have made it work in different ways in practice. Starting with a program theory also allows the evaluator

Box 10.2 Logic models

A logic model is a representation of the relationships between the resources, activities, outputs and outcomes in a project. The logic model makes explicit the rationale behind the design of the project and then how to get from the current state to the desired state. In its simplest form, it describes inputs, actions and outcomes. A logic model for prevention of pressure damage may look like this:

Assessment of peripheral perfusion, mobility and nutrition ⟹ Calculation of risk of pressure ulcer ⟹ Risk mitigated by risk adjusted evidence-based interventions ⟹ Pressure ulcers avoided

The logic model is only as good as each of the assumptions within it. If the assessment is not a good predictor of risk, the ensuing interventions may not be appropriate. If the risk is accurately calculated, but the interventions are not evidence-based or if the wrong interventions for the level of risk are applied, the outcomes may be poor.

Evaluating a pressure ulcer prevention project must look at whether all parts of the assessment were correctly conducted, whether the risk was properly calculated and whether the interventions were appropriate to the risk. If the pressure ulcer rate remains high, this will help to determine whether the issue is compliance with guidance or whether the logic of the project needs to be reviewed.

to trace how the logic of the improvement project evolves over time and which circumstances or contexts influenced that change.

The underlying mechanisms of change triggered by the improvement intervention are rarely perceptible through the senses, and yet they clearly exist, in the same way that love cannot be captured through the five human senses but influences human behaviours. This means that the causes of the improvements are often reconstructed rather than measurable observations and they can still be explored using the perceptions or social constructions, of those involved with and impacted by the improvement. The reliability of these constructions is enhanced by gaining as many different perceptions as possible, including those of patients and managers as well as clinical professionals. Differences in perception are positively helpful, as, rather than giving primacy to the views of one group, the difference can reveal a common mechanism, and 'the juxtaposition of two apparently unrelated matters may give the very first clues to some later insight or explanation' (Spencer et al. 2003, p. 229).

Realist evaluation

Pawson and Tilley (1997) developed a theory-driven evaluation method that they call realist evaluation in response to what they perceived to be a failure of experimental designs of evaluation. They criticised the 'successionist' theory of causality on which experiments are based, which assumes a linear progression of change from status 'a' (before the intervention) to status 'b' (after the intervention) but without explaining how and why the change occurred. Their approach is based on a 'generative' theory of causality, that the intervention does not itself create the change directly but activates people to create it. The approach draws on critical realist philosophy (Bhaskar 2010), which asserts that there are three levels of reality:

1 The *real* level which is the infrastructure and context of action that triggers action
2 The *actual* level in which actions occur (whether observable or not)
3 The *empirical* which is the realm of what is independently (or empirically) observable (Bhaskar 2010)

What happens in any given situation depends on the interplay between the three levels.

The difference between realist and other theory-based evaluation approaches is that a realist program theory specifies in advance what mechanisms will be anticipated to generate the outcomes and what features of the context will affect whether or not those mechanisms operate. Rather than attempt to control for different variables, realist evaluation seeks out and studies the impact of different variables on the predictions to uncover the impact of the context on the actions and therefore the outcomes. Pawson and Tilley (1997) reframed Bhaskar's three levels of reality as:

1 **Context:** What conditions are needed for a measure to trigger mechanisms to produce particular outcomes patterns?
2 **Mechanism:** What does an intervention lead to in order to have a particular outcome in a given context?
3 **Outcomes:** What are the practical effects produced by causal mechanisms being triggered in a given context?

Pawson and Tilley asserted that outcomes are the product of mechanisms that are modified by their context. The mechanisms are the planned causal factors or processes, and, whilst they are not unique to a particular setting, they are triggered only in certain contexts (or are partially triggered in different contexts), and so attention must be paid not only to the intervention but to the context in which it is being implemented. Westhorp (2014) illustrates this by saying that:

> if I am standing on land when I release the tennis ball, gravity will draw it to the ground. If I happen to be underwater, a different mechanism (buoyancy) will cause the ball to float [...] gravity is the stronger force in air and buoyancy the stronger force under water[...] context determines which mechanism "wins" (p. 6)

Designing an evaluation

Theory-driven evaluation is more a way of thinking than a specific method and the design will be dependent on the nature of the question and to some extent the resources available. The black box is agnostic and the methods used to explore it depend on the theories within it:

> All methods can have merit when one puts the theories that can explain a programme at the centre of the evaluation design. No method is seen as the 'gold standard'. Theories should be made explicit, and the evaluation steps should be built around them: by elaborating on assumptions; revealing causal chains; and engaging all concerned parties in this exercise.
>
> (Stame 2004, p. 60)

Whilst it is possible to develop a post hoc program theory (e.g., Dixon-Woods et al. 2011 developed a post hoc theory for the Matching Michigan study), in order to deeply understand the mechanism by which a given outcome is achieved, it is preferable to study the whole journey, not just the outcome. Therefore, ideally the evaluation should be planned and begun before the intervention is implemented.

The first task, therefore, is to surface the assumptions behind the improvement project and make the program theory explicit. It may be necessary to do this at many different levels in order to describe patterns and discrepancies in the assumptions of different stakeholders about how the improvement intervention is expected to work. These assumptions are less likely to be quantifiable and are best uncovered through interview or focus groups, although other qualitative data collection methods (including electronic crowd sourcing) may be appropriate.

The resultant program theory will highlight the anticipated mechanisms of improvement that can then be tested in relation to the specific context under evaluation and the actual outcomes compared against the intended outcomes. For realist evaluations, Pawson and Tilley (1997) suggested that the focus should be on the internal factors that either enhance or inhibit the mechanism rather than searching for an independent variable that might be generalised across all circumstances. They proposed that evaluation is framed in terms of Context-Mechanism-Outcomes (CMO) configurations as propositions of 'what works for whom in which circumstances' (2001, p. 217), which are tested in practice. The program theory is therefore translated into tentative CMO configurations, which direct the design of data collection. The program theory and CMO configurations should consider whether there is a temporal aspect to the improvement and whether the testing will require data to be obtained at different times of the day, days of the week or when different members of staff (or teams) are on duty.

Economic evaluations

For both financial and ethical reasons it is important to establish which interventions add value (the principle of the LEAN approach to improvement is discussed in more detail in Chapter 1). Whilst value refers to more than financial cost, the limits of the budget for health-care services in all countries means it is important for evaluators to consider whether the improvement justifies the cost: whether it is a good return on investment or whether that money might be better spent elsewhere.

Quality improvement interventions may not be cheaper in the short term than current practice; indeed, they might be more expensive but may save money elsewhere in the system. For example, by eliminating poor care that leads to increased length of stay, there might be significant reduction in the cost of an episode of care and there may be saving in the avoidance of a penalty fine or clinical negligence costs.

Airoldi et al. (2014) created a method for assessing how resources should best be deployed through the development of a consensus model that included both social and technical aspects of evaluation. Their model includes a number of dimensions:

- The additional annual funding (the marginal cost) required to run the intervention, compared to current care
- Population health benefit, that is, the number of patients who benefit from the intervention multiplied by the potential benefit in quality
- The extent to which the intervention has the potential to reduce unwarranted variation
- The feasibility: the probability of success (from 0% to 100%) of achieving the assumed benefits in a given context

The model allows each dimension to be assigned a numerical value which can be plotted on a graph to compare different interventions and demonstrate where spending is predicted to add the most value. The model was developed with a wide range of stakeholders to compare different interventions for the same health need and thereby determine the purchasing priorities for healthcare services commissioners. As such, it forms an economic as well as quality evaluation of services.

When evaluating quality improvement projects, it can be challenging to identify absolute costs and in particular cash releasing savings. Healthcare services operate with fixed overhead costs (buildings, supplies and people) and significant change is required to release them. An alternative concept is opportunity costs: the lack of opportunity to use those assets on some other activity or the things that you cannot do if you spend your resources on this chosen process. Evaluation of quality improvement should therefore consider not only what the impact of a given intervention is but also whether outcomes might have been better, if the resources had been used on a different intervention with even more significant impact.

Data sources

As previously discussed, it cannot be assumed that causal factors in social systems are linear and sequential and therefore they may not be repeated or repeatable. A quote that is incorrectly attributed to W. Edwards Deming is 'you can't manage what you can't measure' but in fact what he actually said was:

> It is wrong to suppose that if you can't measure it, you can't manage it – a costly myth. (1994, p. 35)

Social systems are implicitly complex and the interdependence of variables means cause and effect can rarely be demonstrated statistically, and so a standardised data collection protocol may not be the most appropriate. As Deming observed in his theory of Profound Knowledge, quality improvement is dependent on both appreciation of a system and the psychology of change and it follows that a plurality of data sources may be needed.

There is an apparent dichotomy between standardised measurement data and interpretative data, with the former seeking to reduce the data and strip it of its context in order to generalise about probability and interpretative data seeking to specify the impact of context and generalise about theory. The art of a quality improvement evaluator is to find the sweet spot between the two. As Mason (2002) argued:

> different methods and data sources are likely to throw light on different social phenomena or provide different versions or levels of answer to research questions. (p. 190)

Theory-driven evaluation is not based on statistical generalisation and so samples are not subject to considerations of statistical power needed for inferential statistics and nor is it based on controlling for variation through randomisation. Instead, data sources are chosen purposively based on who or what may inform the questions that emerged from the program theory.

Data may be collected from documentary sources, via observation, through interviews and surveys or through secondary analysis of existing datasets (e.g. rates of patient harms), as appropriate to the propositions (or configurations) that emerge from the program theory. The evaluator should be mindful of the burden of evaluation data collection on staff who are also trying to introduce change into the system and how this might influence the integrity and reliability of the data.

Interviews

Interviewing has been described by Burgess (1984, p. 102) as a 'conversation with a purpose'. Realist interviewing is directed toward testing the program theory or as Pawson and Tilley advised, the CMO configuration, by giving respondents the opportunity to confirm, falsify and refine the theory. It is still important to avoid confirmation bias and so respondents should be required to discuss a real life example and to explain how they thought the mechanisms had worked within it. The role of the interviewer is to probe the places where the interviewee diverges from the proposed theory. Interviews might include patients as well as service providers and this juxtaposition of differing views may reveal a deeper mechanism that influences both versions but is triggered in different ways in different contexts.

Weiss (1994) suggested that if the aim is to obtain more than a choice amongst predetermined categories, the requirement that the questions are asked of all the respondents in the same way should be dropped and the respondents should be probed for further explanation or discussion. Responses to a fixed question will elicit a decontextualised or generalised response that is more likely to conform to the generally accepted account and will be less likely to reveal the experience of the local implementation. Bourdieu (1977) agreed and argued that it is by moving from the general to the specific and personal that the actual processes will be revealed. Mason (2002) concurred that an interviewer who is interested in the 'social process that operates situationally' will need to ask:

> situational rather than abstract questions, you will want to take cues from the ongoing dialogue with your interviewees about what to ask them next, rather than go into the interaction entirely pre-scripted. (p. 64)

How the interviews are conducted also needs consideration. Shuy (2002) examined the relative merits of face–to-face and telephone interviews and observed that telephone interviews have a higher response rate than face-to-face interviews and a reduced interviewer effect. On the other hand, interviewers find it harder to probe as there are no non-verbal cues.

Observation

Mays and Pope (1995) noted that observational research is particularly useful for studying the roles played by different people and the relationships between them. Dixon-Woods et al. (2012) have demonstrated the use of 'ethnographic methods' in their studies of the application of a national quality improvement project to study the 'black box'. Through observation, they were able to demonstrate that measuring central line infections is a social process that varies significantly between and within hospitals (see Box 2.3 for further detail).

The extent to which the observer is seen to be independent reflects the philosophical underpinning of the evaluation and the extent to which the evaluator is seeking to measure the impact of a specific variable in a controlled manner. Theory-driven evaluation is looking to gain greater understanding of the process, and Hammersley and Atkinson (1994) argue that:

> all social research is a form of participant observation because we cannot study the social world without being part of it. (p. 249)

McDonald (2005) described a form of observation in which the observer not only participates but asks question in situ. Shadowing is a technique in which the researcher closely follows a member of staff over an extended period and asks questions that will prompt a running commentary with the person being shadowed. Shadowing provides a bridge between observation and interpretation and allows access to concepts that are difficult to articulate and also allows the context of the observation to be captured.

Documentary review

Mason (2002) observed that documents are always constructed by their authors and can therefore provide a contextual background of the authors' views that can frame data collected by other instruments. Marwick (2001) suggested that documents can be examined for the information that the author intended to convey (the 'factual' elements) or for the unintentional or indirect data. However documents are constructed, they can reveal an additional viewpoint. An example of documentary review would be the examination of policies in order to demonstrate how the organisation or unit has considered the improvement intervention and whether it has been embedded in the everyday working.

Surveys

Surveys are useful methods for collecting evaluation data and can be low cost if technology (including on line surveys) is used to distribute and capture the data. This ease means that surveys may be used at a single point in time (cross sectional) or can measure change over time (longitudinal). Surveys can capture differing conditions and outcomes and can measure the perceptions of participants. Surveys do not capture individual differences and thus require a clear conceptualisation of the question to be asked but can provide large volumes of data from which statistical generalisations can be made. As with other methods, the design must clearly relate to the evaluation question and, if used, to the program theory.

Secondary data analysis

Healthcare organisations collect huge amounts of data by a range of methods. Secondary analysis of existing data which was collected for a different purpose can be a useful tool for evaluators as long as the assumptions that drive the inclusion and exclusion criteria are consistent with the evaluation question. A good example of the challenges of secondary analysis is the measurement of hospital mortality. In the United Kingdom, a number of mortality measures are available. They differ on the sampling (100% of admissions or a basket of diagnostic groups), time of death (in-hospital deaths only or deaths up to 30 days after discharge) and expected or unexpected deaths. All of the measures are appropriate to answer some of the evaluation questions but not others. Once again, clarification about the evaluation question and the program theory is important in order to determine which existing data might be useful.

Analysis of data

Pawson and Manzano-Santaella (2012) urged evaluators to ensure that the data is considered as a whole rather than reducing it to themes removed from their context. The analysis should follow the program theory and demonstrate whether the links between the context, the improvement mechanism and the outcome flow in the way predicted by the propositions or configurations. One way to achieve this is to organise the data into matrices around each configuration. Ritchie and Spencer (1994) have developed a five-stage 'Framework' analysis system that uses both a deductive and an inductive approach and which also acknowledges prior propositions and allows for new explanations to emerge from the data. The development of matrices with separate rows for each data source and columns for each dimension ensures that the data is analysed holistically. The presentation of all the data on each proposition in a single chart exposes negative findings or missing data and guards against assumptions from either the program theory or the culture of the practice being taken from granted in the analysis. The data in the matrices are then explored using abductive reasoning, a form of logical inference, which makes the most sense of incomplete data and is informed by existing theory.

All evaluation has limitations, and it is imperative that evaluators are explicit about their methods and the limitations of their findings to allow others to assess the trustworthiness and to inform the refinement of the program theory and inform future evaluations.

Box 10.3 provides a case study of an evaluation of a quality improvement.

Box 10.3 Case study of a quality improvement evaluation

Bridges and Meyer (2007) used an innovation journey approach to their evaluation of the introduction of a new role designed to improve the patient discharge process. Bridges and Meyer suggested that much of the theory around innovations has been developed from studies of clinical practice and technology rather than social processes involved in embedding new work roles. Their study explored the processes by which these roles became embedded and sustained.

(Continued)

Box 10.3 Case study of a quality improvement evaluation (*Continued*)

Using semi-structured interviews with a range of different professions, focus groups and participant observation and documentary analysis, the authors explored how a new role that had appeared to be successful continued to develop in unanticipated ways.

The roles were designed to manage and remove non-clinical obstacles thus reducing patients' length of stay, for example, by eliminating delays in obtaining laboratory results. The study, unusually, commenced 2 years after the roles had been introduced. They found that the roles had become an accepted and valued part of routine practice but that there was a significant difference between their original job description and the work they were doing in practice, demonstrating that an innovation can become institutionalised whilst still establishing and changing its boundaries. Whilst the support workers were still undertaking some of the clerical coordination, they had also taken on the lead in planning and actioning the discharges of the most complex patients. This role had previously only been carried out by registered nurses but had gradually shifted to the new role without any explicit discussion or decision-making. There had been no formal acknowledgement of the shift in the job description and no additional training, leaving the researchers concerned that the standard of care had been compromised.

The shift in the content of the role was a reflection of the complex working environment and pressure on hospital beds. The organisational need to ensure that only the most acutely ill patients were kept in hospital and that no patients were kept on the wards when they were fit enough to be elsewhere meant that the roles, which were introduced to provide administrative support, were directed to other activities. Once the initial effort of introducing the role was completed, the managers turned their attention to new projects and left the role holders to 'get on' with it. The change did not 'stabilise' at this point as had been originally intended and the new role holders gradually took over more aspects of managing the length of stay, until they reached a point at which the relationship between themselves and the ward nurses stabilised. One might have expected the registered nurses to intervene, especially if they thought that the discharges were not being assessed as well when the new role holders took over, but there was no negotiation, and the nurses allowed the change to progress until a stabilisation point was reached.

It remains unclear how the stabilisation point was determined, as the nurses did not perceive that they had influence or responsibility for the quality of the new role holders' input to patient care. Bridges and Meyer concluded that the fact that the new role was charged with a goal, rather than practice process standards, meant that it would inevitably have a more complex and non-linear journey than a more fixed innovation such as a care pathway and they asserted that the parameters of a an improvement project will therefore affect the end point of the change journey. Whilst much previous research has indicated that healthcare practitioners can play an active part in customising innovations for their local utility (e.g., informed by existing informed by existing Ferlie et al. 2005; Locock et al. 2001), Bridges and Meyer (2007) identified contextual attributes (in this case pressure of hospital beds) that constrained managers' and practitioners' abilities to reflect on the role beyond its initial introduction.

Conclusion

Quality Improvement refers to actions designed to continuously enhance the quality of a service rather than to achieve a specific target. Evaluation of quality improvement focuses on trends rather than pre- and post-intervention measurement and seeks to understand the causal factors for improvement in order to inform future activities to bring about further improvement rather than measure compliance with a process.

Evaluation runs through the whole improvement project with formative evaluations taking place during the implementation of a new process and summative evaluation being conducted once the implementation is considered to be stabilised. Summative evaluations form an overall assessment of the impact of an improvement programme and consider whether a change has occurred, the change is an improvement, the change was related to the interventions and the change has been sustained.

The way in which the evaluation is conducted is dependent on the questions or propositions that are being explored. Improvement uses clinical evidence but is heavily dependent on social processes and so is methodologically agnostic. Thus, rather than defining a 'correct' way of conducting evaluation, it is more important to ensure that there is internal consistency between epistemology, methodology and methods (Carter and Little 2007).

The questions or propositions to be evaluated are derived from the program theory and thus it is important to make this explicit. Whilst post hoc program theory can be deduced, theory-driven evaluations take a prospective program theory as their starting point for evaluation design.

In summary, understanding the impact of quality improvement interventions is imperative for the refinement of the design and further improvement. It is only by conducting a robust evaluation that the questions about whether a change is an improvement and was related to the intervention can be properly answered.

References

Airoldi, M., Morton, A., Smith, J.A., and Bevan, G. (2014) STAR – People-powered prioritization a 21st-century solution to allocation headaches. *Medical Decision Making* 34(8): 965–975.

Attaran, M. (2000) Why does reengineering fail? A practical guide for successful implementation. *Journal of Management Development* 19(9): 794–801.

Beer, M. and Nohria, N. (2000) Resolving the tension between theories E and O of change. Breaking the code of change. In: Beer, M., Nohria, N, editors. *Breaking the Code of Change*. Boston, MA: Harvard Business School Press.

Benning, A., Ghaleb, M., Suokas, A., Dixon-Woods, M., Dawson, J., Barber, N. et al. (2011) Large scale organisational intervention to improve patient safety in four UK hospitals: Mixed method evaluation. *British Medical Journal* 342: 195.

Bhaskar, R. (2010) *Reclaiming Reality: A Critical Introduction to Contemporary Philosophy*. London: Taylor & Francis.

Blamey, A. and Mackenzie, M. (2007) Theories of change and realistic evaluation: Peas in a pod or apples and oranges? *Evaluation* 13(4): 439–455.

Bourdieu, P. (1977) *Outline of a Theory of Practice*. Cambridge: Cambridge University Press.

Bridges, J. and Meyer, J. (2007) Policy on new workforce roles: A discussion paper. *International Journal of Nursing Studies* 44(4): 635–644.

Burgess, R.G. (1984) *In the Field: An Introduction to Field Research*. London: Allen and Unwin.

Carter, S.M. and Little, M. (2007) Justifying knowledge, justifying method, taking action: Epistemologies, methodologies, and methods in qualitative research. *Qualitative Health Research* 17(10): 1316–1328.

Chen, Y., Hemming, K., Stevens, A., and Lilford, R. (2016) Secular trends and evaluation of complex interventions: The rising tide phenomenon. *BMJ Quality and Safety* 25(5): 303–310.

Deming, W. (1994) *The New Economics*. Cambridge, MA: Massachusetts Institute of Technology.

Dixon-Woods, M. (2013) The problem of context in quality improvement. In: *Perspectives on Context: A Selection of Essays Considering the Role of Context in Successful Quality Improvement*. London: Health Foundation.

Dixon-Woods, M., Bosk, C., Aveling, E., Goeschel, C., and Pronovost, P. (2011) Explaining Michigan: Developing an ex post theory of a quality improvement program. *Milbank Quarterly* 89(2): 167–205.

Dixon-Woods, M., Leslie, M., Bion, J., and Tarrant, C. (2012) What counts? An ethnographic study of infection data reported to a patient safety program. *Milbank Quarterly* 90(3): 548–591.

Eisenhardt, K.M. (1989) Building theories from case study research. *Academy of Management Review*, 14(4): 532–550.

Ferlie, E., Fitzgerald, L., Wood, M., and Hawkins, C. (2005) The (non) spread of innovations: The mediating role of professionals. *Academy of Management Journal* 48(1): 117–134.

Feynman, R. and Sackett, P. (1985) "Surely You're Joking Mr. Feynman!": Adventures of a curious character. *American Journal of Physics* 53(12): 1214–1216.

Greenhalgh, T., Robert, G., MacFarlane, F., Bate, P., and Kyriakidou, O. (2004) Diffusion of innovations in service organizations: Systematic review and recommendations. *Milbank Quarterly* 82(4): 581–629.

Hammersley, M. and Atkinson, P. (1994) Ethnography and participant observation. In: Denzin, N.K., Lincoln, Y.S, editors. *Handbook of Qualitative Research*. Thousand Oaks, CA: Sage.

Hartley, J.F. (1994) Case studies in organisational research. In: Casewell, C., Symon, G, editors. *Qualitative Methods and Analysis in Organisational Research – A Practical Guide*. London: Sage.

Health Foundation (2011) *Safer Patients Initiative Phase Two: A Controlled Evaluation of the Second Phase of a Complex Patient Safety Intervention Implemented in English Hospitals*. London: Health Foundation.

Kilo, C.M. (1998) A framework for collaborative improvement: Lessons from the Institute for Healthcare Improvement's Breakthrough Series. *Quality Management in Healthcare* 6(4): 1–14.

Kirkpatrick, D. (1976) Evaluation of training. In: Craig, R, editors. *Training and Development Handbook: A Guide to Human Resource Development*. New York, NY: McGraw-Hill.

Lincoln, Y.S. and Guba, E.G. (1985) *Naturalistic Inquiry*. Newbury Park, CA: Sage.

Locock, L., Dopson, S., Chambers, D., and Gabbay, J., (2001) Understanding the role of opinion leaders in improving clinical effectiveness. *Social Science and Medicine* 53(6): 745–757.

Martin, V. (2003) *Leading Change in Health and Social Care*. London: Routledge.

Marwick, A. (2001) *The New Nature of History: Knowledge, Evidence, Language*. Basingstoke: Palgrave.

Mason, J. (2002) *Qualitative Researching*, 2nd edn. London: Sage.

Mayo, E. (1993) *The Human Problems of an Industrial Civilization*. New York, NY: Macmillan.

Mays, N. and Pope, C. (1995) Qualitative research: Rigour and qualitative research. *British Medical Journal* 311(6997): 109–112.

McDonald, S. (2005) Studying actions in context: A qualitative shadowing method for organizational research. *Qualitative Research*, 5(4): 455–473.

Øvretveit, J. (2000) The economics of quality – A practical approach. *International Journal of Health Care Quality Assurance* 13(5): 200–207.

Pawson, R. and Manzano-Santaella, A. (2012) A realist diagnostic workshop. *Evaluation* 18(2): 176–191.

Pawson, R. and Tilley, N. (1997) *Realistic Evaluation*. London: Sage.

Ritchie, J. and Spencer, L. (1994) Qualitative data analysis for applied policy research. In: Bryman, A., Burgess, R.G, editors. *Analyzing Qualitative Data*. London: Routledge, pp. 173–194.

Rittell, H. and Webber, M. (1973) Dilemmas in a general theory of planning. *Policy Sciences* 4: 155–169.

Scriven, M. (1967) *The Methodology of Evaluation Perspectives of Curriculum Evaluation, and AERA monograph Series on Curriculum Evaluation No. 1*. Chicago, IL: Rand McNally.

Self, D.R. and Schraeder, M. (2009) Enhancing the success of organizational change: Matching readiness strategies with sources of resistance. *Leadership and Organization Development Journal* 30(2): 167–182.

Shojania, K. and Grimshaw, J. (2005) Evidence-based quality improvement: The state of the science. *Health Affairs* 24(1): 138–150.

Shuy, R.W. (2002) In person versus telephone interviewing. In: Gubrium, J.F., Holstein, J, editors. *Handbook of Interview Research: Context and Method*. Thousand Oaks, CA: Sage.

Spencer, L., Ritchie, J., and O'Connor, W. (2003) *Qualitative Research Practice: A Guide for Social Science Students and Researchers*. Thousand Oaks, CA: Sage.

Stame, N. (2004) Theory-based evaluation and types of complexity. *Evaluation* 10(1): 58–76.

Van de Ven, A., Polley, D., Garud, R., and Venkatamaran, S. (1999) *The Innovation Journey*. Oxford: Oxford University Press.

Weiss, C. (1995) Nothing as practical as good theory: Exploring theory-based evaluation for comprehensive community initiatives for children and families. In: Connell, J.P., Kubisch, A.C., Schorr, L.B., Weiss, C.H, editors. *New Approaches to Evaluating Community Initiatives: Volume 1, Concepts, Methods, and Contexts*. Washington, DC: The Aspen Institute.

Weiss, R.S. (1994) *Learning from Strangers: The Art and Method of Qualitative Interview Studies*. New York, NY: Free Press.

Werkman, R.A. (2009) Understanding failure to change: A pluralistic approach and five patterns. *Leadership and Organization Development Journal* 30(7): 664–684.

Westhorp. (2014) *Realist Impact Evaluation: An Introduction*. London: Overseas Development Institute. Available from: www.odi.org/sites/odi.org.uk/files/odi-assets/publications-opinion-files/9138.pdf (accessed on 25 September 2016).

Index